Chronic Pain: a Handbook for N~~urses~~

This book is due for return on or before the last date shown below.

Chronic Pain:
a Handbook for Nurses

Marcus Munafò MA(Oxon), MSc, PhD

and

Jacquie Trim RGN

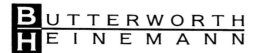
BUTTERWORTH
HEINEMANN

OXFORD   AUCKLAND   BOSTON   JOHANNESBURG   MELBOURNE   NEW DELHI

Butterworth-Heinemann
Linacre House, Jordan Hill, Oxford OX2 8DP
225 Wildwood Avenue, Woburn, MA 01801-2041
A division of Reed Educational and Professional Publishing Ltd

℞ A member of the Reed Elsevier plc group

First published 2000

British Library Cataloguing in Publication Data
A catalogue record for this book is available from the British Library

Library of Congress Cataloguing in Publication Data
A catalogue record for this book is available from the Library of Congress

ISBN 0 7506 4120 7

Typeset by E & M Graphics, Midsomer Norton, Bath
Printed and bound by MPG Books Ltd, Bodmin, Cornwall

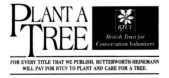

Contents

Contributors

D. J. Dalgleish MA, MB, FRCS, FRCA
Specialist Registrar in Anaesthesia, Wessex School of Anaesthesia

C. Duncombe RGN, BSc (Hons) Nursing Studies, PGCEA
Clinical Nurse Specialist, Hospital Palliative Care Team, Southampton
University Hospitals NHS Trust

J. F. Hazelgrove BSc, MB BS, FRCA
Specialist Registrar in Anaesthetics, Southampton General Hospital

G. T. Lewith MA, DM, MRCP, MRCGP
Honorary Senior Research Fellow, Honorary Consultant Physician,
University Department of Medicine, Southampton General Hospital

M. Munafò MA (Oxon), MSc, PhD
Research Fellow, Imperial Cancer Research Fund General Practice
Research Group, Institute of Health Sciences, University of Oxford

V. M. Norris RGN
Chronic Pain Nurse, Southampton University Hospitals NHS Trust;
formerly Neurosciences Staff Nurse, Wessex Neurological Centre,
Southampton

K. Penn RGN, BSc(Hons), Onc. Cert.
Formerly Clinical Nurse Specialist, Hospital Palliative Care Team,
Southampton University Hospitals NHS Trust

P. Pitcher RGN, MSc Psychosocial Palliative Care
Clinical Nurse Specialist, Hospital Palliative Care Team, Southampton
University Hospitals NHS Trust

C. Price MB BCh, DCh, FRCA
Consultant in Anaesthesia and Pain Relief, Southampton General
Hospital

M. Stuart Taylor BSc, MB BS, FFARCS
Consultant Anaesthetist and Lead Consultant for the Acute Pain Service,
Southampton General Hospital

S. Thomas RGN, ENB 219, ENB 998
Acting Charge Nurse, Orthopaedics, Southampton General Hospital

J. Trim RGN
Acute Pain Sister, Southampton General Hospital

Preface

This book is designed to introduce to an overview of theories of chronic pain, types of chronic pain, its assessment and management, and the role of specialist services in chronic pain. Although primarily intended to be read by an audience of practising nurses who are likely to come into contact with patients with chronic pain during the course of their work, it will be of interest to other health professionals and students for whom chronic pain is a relevant area.

That chronic pain is a relevant issue for the majority of health professionals is made clear by the scale of the problem. A substanstial proportion of the patients that any health professional will come into contact with will suffer from some problem of chronic pain, and this may or may not be related to the reason for which the health professional is seeing the patient. An awareness, therefore, of the various types of chronic pain that exist, as well as the causes that may underlie these, allied to an appreciation of what treatments the patient may already be undergoing or may in future benefit from, is essential to good practice. In particular, an awareness of the extent to which a chronic pain problem may have an impact on other areas of a patient's life will allow a much clearer understanding of an individual patient's needs.

The book may roughly be divided into two halves. The first half covers theoretical issues, types of chronic pain and the role of specialist services. Chapter 1 discusses the basic science of pain, in particular the physiology and anatomy, while Chapter 2 covers assessment and discusses the problems associated with attempting to quantify an entity for which no direct measure exists. Chapters 3, 5 and 6 address the various types of chronic pain problems that exist, in particular chronic pain syndromes and the important distinction between malignant and non-malignant chronic pain. Finally, Chapter 4 outlines the functions served by a typical pain clinic.

The second half of the book is concerned with the pain management techniques that are available, including alternative treatments for which there is substantial or growing evidence of support. Chapter 8 outlines the basic pharmacological options available, while Chapter 9 describes the use of psychological and behavioural techniques in the management of chronic pain. Alternative treatments are discussed in the final three chapters, including transcutaneous electrical nerve stimulation (TENS) in

Chapter 10, acupuncture in Chapter 11, and relaxation and hypnosis in Chapter 12.

Throughout the book the emphasis is on a multi-disciplinary and multi-method understanding of chronic pain and a similarly holistic approach to the management of chronic pain. The value of pharmacological approaches to the management of chronic pain is clear, but this has its limitations. The use of psychological, behavioural and other management techniques is gaining in popularity as it becomes clear that a broader approach that encompasses these alternatives will provide relief to a far greater number of patients. Many of these alternative methods have the advantage of being cheap and easy to learn by the patient, requiring minimal supervision after an initial period of training, in keeping with modern themes of empowerment and patient choice.

M. Munafò and J. Trim

1
Anatomy and physiology of pain

D. J. Dalgleish

Introduction

The traditional view of pain is that tissue damage sends messages directly from the periphery to the brain via clearly identifiable pathways. It has also been held that the more intense the tissue damage then the more severe is the pain. This theory of pain would suggest that if the connections were to be severed then the message would not be transmitted. The nervous system could then, in the past, have been thought of as a telephone exchange having fixed connections between where the tissue damage occurs and the specific parts of the nervous system where the pain is felt.

It is now accepted that this concept of direct transmission of pain is not complete. There is layer upon layer of complexity involved. At its simplest, definite channels for transmission of painful nerve impulses do exist and these may suffice to describe how 'physiological pain' is felt. Physiological pain involves noxious stimuli briefly activating peripheral nociceptors (see below). This has a clear protective function and is thus beneficial to the organism. The types of condition managed in pain clinics, however, are highly complex and the mechanisms involved are not yet completely understood. In this 'pathological pain' the signals transmitted may be modified at every level, from the peripheral receptors through the peripheral nerves to the spinal cord and brain. What is more, the pain process itself may affect the neurones that transmit the pain. Whereas the nervous system was once seen in much the same way as a collection of fixed wires, it is now known to be highly changeable, or plastic. In certain circumstances even a brief noxious stimulus may have far-reaching effects in the development of a chronic pain syndrome.

It is well known that there is a wide spectrum of pain states between, at one extreme, a patient who denies pain but has severe tissue damage (e.g. on a battlefield) and at the other a patient who may have been denied a diagnosis but is debilitated by chronic pain. The diagnosis and treatment of these latter patients can be most difficult and requires a knowledge of the many types and mechanisms of pain discussed in this book, and the corresponding management techniques. This chapter attempts to provide a basic concept of the anatomical pathways and physiology of pain.

Pain receptors

Pain receptors (nociceptors) are naked endings of Aδ and C nerve fibres. Through them, the body is able to detect the occurrence, location, intensity and duration of noxious stimuli, and thereby signal pain sensation. These pain receptors are widespread in the superficial layers of the skin, and also certain internal tissues such as the periosteum, joint surfaces, skeletal muscle and tooth pulp. Most of the other deep tissues are not richly supplied with pain receptors, but widespread tissue damage can cause aching pain in these areas.

Broadly, there are two categories of pain receptor: There are those that respond to mechanical deformation and those that respond to a wide range of adverse stimuli including chemical, thermal and mechanical stimuli.

The first group of receptors where intense mechanical stimulation leads directly to nerve endings being activated causes the sensation of pain to be conducted by the Aδ fibres (see below).

Injury also releases chemicals and neurotransmitters such as substance P, histamine, bradykinin and prostaglandins, all of which may interact to activate pain-sensitive C fibres.

- **Substance P**. A peptide neurotransmitter that is released locally from the nerve endings. It is depleted from the nerve fibres by capsaicin – one of the active ingredients in chilli peppers. This is the explanation for the heat and pain experienced in the mouth during a hot curry and, afterwards, its relative insensitivity.
- **Histamine**. An amine that is released from mast cells; it also has a significant role to play in anaphylaxis when released systemically.
- **Bradykinin**. A small, short-lived, peptide that is produced from precursor molecules and is destroyed by angiotensin converting enzyme with a half-life of only a few seconds. Together, histamine and bradykinin are responsible for the local tissue swelling, redness and pain (three of the cardinal signs of inflammation – in Latin turgor, rubor and dolor).
- **Prostaglandins**. These are unsaturated fatty acid derived from arachidonic acid in the cell membrane. Non-steroidal anti-inflammatory drugs (including aspirin) inhibit prostaglandin production thus giving rise to their analgesic effect.

Ascending pathways

The detection of the threatened or actual tissue damage is transmitted by the receptors to the nervous system along certain types of nerve fibres called Aδ and C fibres. The classification of nerve fibres is primarily to do with their size and whether or not they are surrounded by a coating of myelin, which is a lipid. Myelination serves to insulate and speed up the conduction of impulses along the nerve. 'A' fibres are all myelinated but fall into four partly overlapping groups, α, β, γ, δ, in decreasing order of size. 'C' fibres are unmyelinated.

The Aδ fibres, which are thinly insulated with myelin, rapidly transmit this signal of tissue damage to the central nervous system. The smaller C fibres are responsible for the secondary pain – this is the uncomfortable sensation that starts after the sharp initial pain and then persists. The Aδ fibres transmit signals at approximately 10 m/s compared to the slower C fibres at 1–2 m/s. Therefore, after a tall man stubs his toe, the initial sharp, well-localized pain (Aδ fibre activity) is felt significantly before the persistent aching (C fibre activity).

The peripheral nerves have well described anatomic courses through the body to the central nervous system. These sensory nerves have their cell bodies in a swelling on the posterior root (dorsal root ganglion) of the spinal nerve on each side and then enter the spinal cord. The nerve fibres synapse (transmit their messages to other nerve fibres) in the dorsal horn, and it is here that much of the modulation of pain transmission occurs.

The majority of the nerve fibres carrying the pain impulses then cross the midline of the cord and ascend as the spinothalamic tract. This is a group of fibres that pass from the spine to the thalamus – a structure that sits underneath the cerebral hemispheres. There are other named tracts that carry pain sensation travelling up the spinal cord to various parts of the central nervous system. Some of these stay on the side that the pain was detected (ipsilateral tracts), while others cross the midline (contralateral tracts).

The signals that are transmitted by the Aδ fibres end up by actually being felt and experienced in very specific areas of the surface of the brain (the sensory cortex). Here, there is a map of the surface of the body with more attention being paid (i.e. a greater number of neurones) to sensitive areas that are well innervated (e.g. the thumb) than to less sensitive areas (e.g. the back). This pathway allows both rapid detection and localization of the site of potential injury. The burning secondary pain carried by the C fibres has a much wider distribution in the brain and is therefore less easily localized. It also probably accounts for the profound emotional aspects of chronic pain.

Descending pathways

As well as pain pathways that ascend from the peripheries via the spinal cord to the brain there are other nerve fibres that descend from the brain and affect the transmission, and hence the sensation, of the pain. This modulation of the pain may occur anywhere but happens especially in the early synapses in the dorsal horn of the spinal cord. Pharmacological agents can likewise be effective analgesics at many points on the nerve pathways of pain, both to and from the brain.

Better understanding of these mechanisms of pain requires knowledge of the role of the previously described ascending pathways and the complexity of descending inhibitory or facilitatory influences affecting the signal.

The cerebral aqueduct is a narrow canal in the midbrain that connects the third ventricle (part of the thalamus) to the fourth ventricle (between the cerebellum and the pons and medulla).

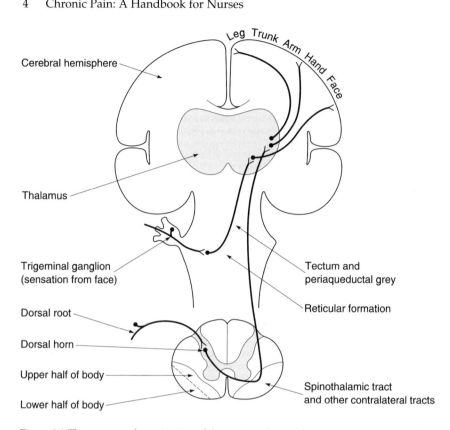

Figure 1.1 The course and termination of the main pathways for pain and temperature, i.e. the spinothalamic tract

The grey matter surrounding the aqueduct (the periaqueductal grey – PAG) and many other parts of the brain stem (e.g. the raphe nuclei) can activate descending pathways. These pathways can inhibit the nociceptive stimulus, probably at dorsal horn levels. They contain many nerves that use 5-hydroxytryptamine (5HT, also known as serotonin) as their neurotransmitter. Other descending pathways are reliant upon noradrenaline (NA). Both 5HT and NA are described as monoamines. Direct electrical stimulation of the PAG and raphe nuclei causes analgesia and, in addition, the cerebral cortex can influence these descending monoaminergic pathways in complex ways.

This control of the transmission of pain from the peripheries to where it is sensed in the brain is believed to occur because of inhibition of the chemical mediators of nociceptive activation. It occurs through liberation of various types of neurotransmitters – the action of many of which can be modified by drugs.

The endogenous opiate-like peptides (endorphins) are one group of chemicals that decrease the transmission of the pain signal in the dorsal horn. Opioid receptors also exist in the brain and the peripheral nerves.

Narcotic analgesics such as morphine will mimic the effect of the endorphins in the central nervous system, but will also affect opioid receptors elsewhere in the body, causing many side-effects.

Other drugs, which at present are used less commonly than opioids, can also have profound effects by acting in the region of the dorsal horn. Ketamine exerts its powerful analgesic effect via NMDA (N-methyl D aspartate) receptors. There are various stimulants that are widely used in veterinary anaesthesia and are being introduced as agents for pain relief in humans.

Gate control theory

In its simplest form, this theory suggests that the dorsal horn of the spinal cord acts as a gate for the control of painful sensations into the ascending neurones. The activity in the Aδ and C fibres keeps this gate open and activation of the larger myelinated Aβ fibres closes the gate. This is accomplished via inhibitory interneurones excited by the Aβ, fibres which decrease the transmission from the C fibres upwards to the brain. The gating principle provides an elegant explanation for some well-known phenomena, for instance the tendency to rub a sore spot to alleviate the pain. Theoretically, rubbing the skin will activate large myelinated Aβ fibres, which will close the gate. A similar mechanism may underlie the perceived effects of such therapies as acupuncture and TENS. The descending pathways previously mentioned may also work by closing the gating mechanism.

Referred pain

Referred pain is said to occur when the pain that is sensed is displaced from its true source in an internal organ and felt on the surface of the body. The pain is not usually referred to the skin overlying the organ but to an area that is innervated by the same spinal cord segment as the organ. For instance, pain in the shoulder region (C3–C4) may be caused by irritation of the diaphragm.

The probable explanation is that pain fibres from a particular organ synapse with the same part of the spinal cord as do the nerves from the relevant area of skin. The brain is not used to interpreting messages from the internal organs and so may mistake this nervous activity as coming from the associated area of skin.

Changes in the nervous system

Allodynia is pain due to a stimulus that would not normally provoke pain. An example of this is the painful feeling of a warm shower on sunburnt skin.

Hyperalgesia is an increased response to a stimulus that is normally painful. Hyperalgesia may be felt either at the site of the injury or at

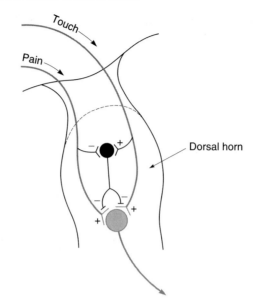

Figure 1.2 The gate control theory of pain: activity in small C fibres (pain) would keep the gate open, whereas impulses reaching the dorsal horn through large A fibres in the medial portion of the dorsal root would close the gate. Although the gate control hypothesis has been severely criticized in recent years, it has stimulated much research and the development of therapeutic devices for pain control. *Black*, inhibitory interneurone; *grey*, primary afferent fibres and spinal projection neurone. (After Melzack, R. and Wall, P. D. (1965) Pain mechanisms: a new theory. *Science* 150, 971–9)

nearby undamaged tissue. It is caused by two main mechanisms. First, it occurs with sensitization of the peripheral nociceptors by locally released chemical mediators of inflammation. For example, if you have an infected toe, it will be more painful if you stub it against a wall than it would otherwise be. Hyperalgesia also occurs because of changes in the level of activation of the nerve cells in the spinal cord.

This leads to the important phenomenon in chronic pain called 'wind up'. The neurones in the dorsal horn can exist in various states of readiness to transmit their message to the brain. It is possible to partially activate them (to wind them up) so that a small further stimulation may tip them over the edge into firing. This state of 'wind up' may mean that not only is a painful sensation transmitted at a lower threshold than it would have been before but also sensations from a wide area surrounding the perceived area of tissue damage may be interpreted as pain. Importantly, it can also mean that signals from nerves that are carrying non-noxious sensations may be wrongly interpreted as pain by the CNS. Aβ fibres carry the sensation of touch from the peripheries but if nerve cells in the dorsal horn are sufficiently wound up then the messages from the Aβ fibres may be transmitted as pain signals.

Wind up will occur to a greater or lesser extent following all injuries. However, it may be particularly important following long-term peripheral nociceptor activation (e.g. degenerative back disease) or following damage to nerves themselves which leads to abnormal messages being transmitted.

Types of chronic pain

Nociceptive

Persistent activation of peripheral nociceptors is a significant factor in many chronic pain states, both malignant and non-malignant. For instance, in chronic rheumatoid arthritis inflammatory mediators will constantly stimulate the free nerve endings of the Aδ and C fibres. Stimulation produces a signal that travels to the dorsal horn of the spinal cord. It may then be widely distributed to many areas of the brain and spinal cord. Therapy directed against the cause of the pain may be possible in chronic nociceptive pain unlike many other types of chronic pain.

Neuropathic

When neural tissue is damaged, its function necessarily alters. Damage to nerves that carry pain may lead to severe chronic pain states. This may occur in both the peripheries and the central nervous system. The injury may be obvious; for example, chronic pain may develop in surgical scars (mastectomy, thoracotomy). Alternatively, it may be microscopic, such as the neuropathic pain after herpes infection. This type of chronic pain may even be felt in limbs years after they have been amputated (phantom limb pain). Damage to the spinal cord or cerebrovascular accidents may also be responsible for such pain.

   The abnormal function of the nerves themselves means that the patient actually feels pain as if the nociceptors were being activated, when in fact they are not. The management of neuropathic pain includes the use of drugs that are not usually thought of as analgesics. Examples include anti-epileptic drugs, which tend to damp down unwanted activity in neurones, and antidepressants, such as amitriptyline.

Complex regional pain syndrome

'Reflex sympathetic dystrophy' and 'causalgia' are now classified as complex regional pain syndromes (CRPS) I and II respectively. They are incompletely understood entities from the physiological and anatomical point of view and consist of a constellation of symptoms and signs including pain, changes in the soft tissues and bones, and an element of dysfunction of the autonomic nervous system. CRPS are often considered to be a type of neuropathic pain. Peripherally, it has been suggested that the nociceptors may become sensitive to noradrenaline (to which they are usually insensitive) and the sympathetic nervous system somehow maintains the state of pain. Centrally, a state of significant wind up occurs which lowers the threshold for painful stimuli. Hence part of the treatment includes guanethidine, which depletes the nerve terminals of noradrenaline and clonidine which may act to reduce its release.

Conclusion

All classifications are subject to error, and real life reflects this. In an individual patient there may be multiple explanations for a chronic pain state and, therefore, concentrating on just one aspect of cause and effect is rarely helpful in the long run. There is a complex interplay between the neurological description of the pain and the psychological state of the patient experiencing it.

Pre-emptive analgesia

A transient injury, such as surgery, initiates the central sensitization known as wind up. However, this hypersensitive state itself outlasts the duration of the injury. It has been proposed that if the injury is pre-empted by analgesia then the wind up will be lessened or it may even fail to occur. It is clear that the surgical insult has two phases, the first during the actual tissue damage and the second during the phase of inflammation before tissue healing. Both of these phases have the potential to initiate central sensitization and, therefore, both must be blocked to constitute effective pre-emptive analgesia. Attacking the pain at a variety of levels provides the best analgesia. Non-steroidal anti-inflammatory drugs will exert their effect on peripheral sensitization of nociceptors. Local anaesthetic infiltration and nerve blocks will prevent transmission of the stimulus centrally. Opioids and other analgesics such as paracetamol and ketamine have their effect mainly at the spinal cord level. As yet there is not any firm proof that pre-emptive analgesia has any clinical advantages but further studies are warranted.

Pathophysiology associated with pain

The physiology concerning the transmission of pain has been briefly outlined. However, the control of pain is not only necessary for humanitarian reasons – pain itself will tend to cause various patho-physiological disturbances in the body, and is a significant contributory factor in subsequent morbidity.

Pain is an important factor in increasing the neuroendocrine stress response. The effects of the increased sympathetic drive include tachycardia and hypertension, both of which may prove to be detrimental to the patient. At the same time, pain in the thorax or abdomen will impair lung expansion and so further decrease the amount of oxygen available for vital processes. Delays to postoperative mobilization will not only increase the risks of deep vein thrombosis but will also increase hospital stay and costs.

Summary
- The pathways involved in pain transmission and perception are not fixed but are changeable. They sometimes change permanently because of the messages transmitted.
- Specialized receptors pass messages to the neurones carrying pain. These nerve cells then connect with higher centres in various parts of the central nervous system.
- The way that pain is perceived is affected both by messages descending from the brain and by other peripheral stimulation.
- Pain can be referred from an internal organ to a distant site.
- Chronic pain states are characterized by alterations in the way the nervous system perceives the pain from the receptor level to the higher centres.
- Analgesia that is supplied early (sometimes even before the insult occurs) and is aimed at many of the different levels where pain is processed may provide the best relief.
- Pain can have important deleterious effects on many aspects of the body's normal functioning and repair processes.

Bibliography

1. Miller, R. D. (ed.) (1999) *Anaesthesia*, 4th edn. Edinburgh: Churchill Livingstone.
2. Heimer, R. (1995) *The Human Brain and Spinal Cord*. New York/Berlin: Springer Verlag.
3. Sinnatamby, C. S. (1999) *Last's Anatomy*, 10th edn. Edinburgh: Churchill Livingstone.
4. Dray, A. (1995) Inflammatory mediators. *British Journal of Anaesthesia*, 75 (2), 125–31.
5. Pocketts, S. (1995) Spinal cord plasticity and chronic pain. *Anaesthesia and Analgesia*, 80 (1), 173–9.
6. Woolf, C. J. and Chong, M. S. (1993) Preemptive analgesia. *Anaesthesia and Analgesia*, 77 (2), 362–79.
7. Walker, S. M. and Cousins, M. J. (1997) Complex regional pain syndromes. *Anaesthesia and Intensive Care*, 25 (2), 113, 125.

2

Assessment of pain

V. M. Norris

Introduction

Chronic pain is quite different, separate and distinct from acute pain. By definition, acute pain is short-lived and acts as a warning to us that harm is present; it is an event that has a foreseeable conclusion. Chronic pain is more than an acute pain that has failed to end; it is a situation, rather than event. It can be perceived by patients as an everlasting experience that serves no useful purpose. Chronic pain is not life-threatening, but the quality of the patient's life may be severely affected. It may affect relationships with partners and spouses, and with family and friends. The chronic pain sufferer may experience sleep disturbances, weight gain, loss of appetite and loss of libido. Patients with chronic pain may also encounter problems with their employment and job loss; this will lead to anxieties about finances and may have a bearing on issues such as leisure activities (i.e., cost implications). When you consider the influence that chronic pain can have on a person's life, and the extent to which it can effect all aspects of life and living, the size of the problem becomes apparent. The potentials for emotional, psychological and behavioural difficulties are clear. Importantly, pain should not be assessed as the sole element of this condition; ideally, assessment of chronic pain should encompass all of these factors. This chapter will consider the nurse's role in the assessment of chronic pain, and the principles of chronic pain assessment. The use of assessment tools for chronic pain will be reflected on and the usefulness and suitability of these tools in an acute setting will be evaluated.

Definitions: assessment and pain

Look through any book, publication or journal about pain, and they will all almost certainly agree that no exact definition of pain seems to exist. This seems incredible when one considers how much literature is available on the subject. This compounds the difficulties that exist when trying to assess pain adequately. What should we be assessing if no adequate definition exists? It would be logical to surmise that the starting point or framework on which to build pain assessment would be the definition of the problem or condition that you are faced with. What then is assessment?

Assessment can be described as an evaluating process of something or someone. Assessment suggests wide-ranging, critical observation and surveillance. It implies the development of a decision-making process and is a systematic collection of information. This process must be continuous and open to further analysis if it is to be of value.

Can pain be defined at all? The most frequently referred to definition is that of the International Association for the Study of Pain:

> Pain is an unpleasant sensory and emotional experience associated with actual or potential tissue damage or described in terms of such damage.[1]

This definition seems to make the task of pain assessment even more complex. It identifies pain as a subjective experience that could be classed as impossible to measure, as there are no 'units' of pain. Pain is felt differently by every patient, and even those with the same or similar conditions will describe pain differently. Combine with this the fact that all nurses are individuals, and will complete pain assessments with different experiences, values, beliefs and ideas guiding this assessment. The potential for variability and numerous misunderstandings is immense. In this situation there is a place for pain scales and assessment tools.

Pain assessment in the Chronic Pain Clinic and the acute ward

Generally speaking, pain is seen as a symptom that has a cause; it needs investigating and the cause of the pain needs treating. The patients seen in a Chronic Pain Clinic do not fall into this straightforward category. Patients who attend a Pain Clinic have pain that persists, usually in excess of three months, although this can vary across individuals. They may continue to feel pain long after conventional treatment has been completed; treatment may cure or modify the medical condition, but not the pain. Some people continue to experience pain after all healing has taken place, or they may continue to feel the pain even though no diagnosis is made or no abnormality is found. Therefore, the philosophy of a Chronic Pain Clinic is not to investigate, treat and cure, but to recognize that the pain is serving no useful purpose and that it is appropriate and necessary to simply treat the pain. These patients will also present to the acute hospital services and be admitted to general wards, as well as Chronic Pain Clinics. The patient's past experiences with the health services can yield a wealth of information about the history of the pain and may reveal the patient's confidence (or lack of it) with the 'system'. Increasing the patient's confidence and trust in the service can be a therapeutic intervention of its own merit.

In a Chronic Pain Clinic environment, patients with long-term pain may need several visits for their pain to be fully assessed. Even then the assessor (be they doctor, nurse or physiotherapist) may feel that they never quite grasp the extreme impact chronic pain has on an individual patient, their life and the lives of those closest to that person. However, if a patient with chronic pain is admitted to an acute clinical area, extensive pain assessment is also required, as in a Pain Clinic. On a busy ward, is this possible, given the demands on nursing time? Difficulties in chronic pain assessment are immediately apparent. As chronic pain has a potential for impact in every part of a person's life, the pain must be assessed wholly and completely with regard to all the different aspects of daily life involved.

The role of the nurse

There are several aspects encompassing the nurse's role in the assessment of chronic pain. The element of assessment cannot be taken in isolation: the role is a combination of coordination, communication and liaison. There is a desperate need to coordinate care and improve lines of communication for patients with chronic pain. Most patients with chronic pain have visited many different departments and clinics, and many people have been involved in their care, maybe some inappropriately. An important role of the nurse is to try to recover some of the patient's confidence in the health care services, which at this point may well be diminished. Ideally, one nurse should oversee the coordination of treatment and act as a point of contact. During the admission, the resulting improvement of organization and communication can only benefit the patient.

Practically, the role also includes ongoing assessment from admission to discharge. For the duration of the admission nurses can, by assessment, identify the need for changes to treatment plans, and implement the changes that are suggested or prescribed by medical staff. Nurses spend the most time with the patient whilst they are inpatients, and so observe and assess the patient for longer periods than other health professionals. They are well used to working as part of a team and so, if other nursing staff are involved in the patient's care, they too will observe and report changes. Other members of the multidisciplinary team will focus on varying aspects of the patient's care. For example, medical staff may focus on the optimal medical or surgical outcome and physiotherapists may concentrate on functional ability. It is to be hoped that through full and comprehensive assessment the nurse will identify the patient's aims of treatment and assist them to achieve their targets.

Obstacles to pain assessment

By far the most important issue when considering pain assessment is believing the patient. The pain must be viewed from the patient's perspective. An empathetic approach to understanding how this pain is affecting this person goes a long way to beginning to gain the trust of someone with chronic pain. This viewpoint is difficult to achieve in that both the patient and the nurse bring their own perspectives and responses to the assessment situation. Both are hampered by previous experiences. The patient's description of his or her discomfort could be affected by the nurse's understanding of pain based on his or her personal and professional beliefs and judgements (i.e. comparing patients with similar or the same conditions). There is great potential for bias and the nurse has to be aware of this. Identifying this tendency and acting accordingly will improve the standard of nursing that the patient receives. There is a now famous definition of pain that encompasses the essence of chronic pain assessment:

> Pain is whatever the patient says it is, and exists when he says it does.[2]

It also, of course, implies that those in the health care professions do not always believe the patient. Believing what the patient tells you is an essential component of chronic pain management. Many patients with a diagnosis of chronic pain follow very similar paths. Imagine a patient in the following scenario.

The patient has suffered a relatively minor injury, insult or illness, but does not improve as expected. The patient sees various doctors and specialists in search of a cure, a diagnosis or a label for their condition. There are repeated investigations, which may show minor abnormalities or be completely normal, for which no specific surgery or treatment is indicated. Someone has probably said that it is 'psychological' and 'is all in your mind' (without full explanation of how this can be). The patient feels angry, distrustful and failed by every doctor and nurse that has been seen.

Now, imagine that you are meeting this patient for the first time and making an assessment. How conducive to a good nursing outcome (i.e., pain relief) is your scepticism of this patient's description of their pain?

Why is it important to assess pain?

As mentioned earlier, pain (and especially chronic pain) is a complex phenomenon. Pain assessment should be classed as an essential requirement when a patient is admitted with this problem. This may reveal problems related to the pain that can be successfully treated, even if the pain itself cannot. For example, such problems may include sleep disturbances, for which an adjuvant drug such as amitriptyline may be indicated; this has a direct pain action and its main side-effect is sleepiness, which can be harnessed for beneficial effect. Good pain assessment is also vital to avoid extreme situations. For example, some nurses may give analgesia routinely during the drug round, while others may wait until the patient requests painkillers before giving analgesia. This is unhelpful in that individual members of nursing staff may administer analgesia in varying patterns to the same patient. Standardizing the assessment process and, therefore, the administration of analgesics could result in improved pain control for patients. Taking this on a step further and using continuing assessment improves the patient's chance of getting continuing improvement in their symptoms.

Assessment helps the nurse to form objectives for planning care and helps identify nursing and medical interventions which may be useful. Subsequent, post-treatment assessments can then be made against a solid baseline, and improvements or deterioration can be identified. Further action can then be implemented immediately. Appraisal enables nursing staff to target the pain with suitable management; this may save time and be more efficient by not using inappropriate treatment. It is important to realize that though the medical and nursing staff by assessing the patient can identify goals, the patient will almost certainly have their own aims and objectives. These may be completely different from the doctor's expectations and different again from the nurse's ideas of satisfactory outcome. Through assessment the patient's goals and aims are highlighted. It is therefore important to ask what the patient's expectations are, to explore whether they are realistic, and whether everyone concerned is working together or independently. A clear, written record of the assessment is important so that good communication can exist between the various health professionals and the patient. A standardized tool for the assessment of pain can help to abolish the potential problem of bias by the nurse.

What should be included in chronic pain assessment?

On admission (or very shortly after) a history is usually taken from the patient by the nurse, in order to identify nursing problems. A pain rating scale should be used on admission to identify a baseline for intensity of pain. The same scale must then be used by all staff at every assessment or enquiry, including non-nursing staff. For someone with chronic pain their other problems will swiftly become apparent, but these details below should definitely be included:

- history (i.e. what started the pain)
- duration
- intensity
- location/site
- extent of pain (i.e., whole leg, whole arm etc.)
- quality of the pain (i.e., description of the pain)
- related symptoms
- disability
- impact on life
- mood
- aggravating/relieving factors
- medication
- all previous treatments

Although this looks like a long list, most of the information can be elicited in a few minutes of conversation. A few simple questions can give abundant information. This may include such enquiries as:

'How did this pain start?'

This question will probably be answered by giving information about the pain history and its duration.

'What is it like, can you describe it?'

This will give information about the quality of the pain, its location, its extent and whether it is constant or intermittent.

'How does it restrict you?'

This question will give indicators about the impact on the patient's daily living and how the patient's relatives/partner or both are affected. The patient may also talk about employment problems and the quality of life they are experiencing.

'What treatments have you tried?'

This is vital to ask, and most patients will have no difficulty remembering, usually because the interventions have not helped them.

'What helps?'

Even though this may seem like an odd question, some people have developed their own routines and methods of pain relief to help themselves a little. The use of complementary therapies is becoming more generally accepted, and these are widely used in chronic conditions. It is important to note anything that has helped. A seemingly small detail, such as the patient describing that rubbing the painful area helps, might indicate that TENS (Transcutaneous Electrical Nerve Stimulation) may be extremely helpful. This would be a critical detail to miss.

The questions shown here do not form part of a formal pain assessment tool. It should be noted that all nurses will ask these questions slightly differently whilst maintaining a theme. The use of an assessment tool is recommended for the way it ensures that the different nurses with their individual approaches assess the same patient in the same way.

After treatment or intervention assessment needs to include the following:

- pain intensity (use the same scale as on admission)
- record of medication/intervention used
- extent of pain
- level of consciousness
- time(s) of assessment
- adverse effects of treatments
- observations, BP, pulse, respirations

Observational pain assessment

Nurses are highly skilled at observing patients and identifying problems, and so this method of assessment should be highly valued. It is also quick and simple to do. Simply observe the patient and record what you see. These are some examples, though there are many more than are listed here:

- what is mobility like?
- does the patient limp?
- do they use a stick/crutches/their partner for support?
- does the patient favour one side of their body?
- do they hold/protect/rub an area of their body?
- does the patient groan/moan/gasp on movement?
- is the patient withdrawn and tearful or chatty and cheerful?

These observations provide the nurse with information that will supplement what may have already been identified. Observation is not to be used instead of full assessment but, rather, complements it.

Pain assessment tools

A pain assessment tool is essential for the uniform collection of information. Different nurses will be involved in nursing care, and so this consistency is vital in ensuring continuity. There are many different pain assessment tools, which fall into two main categories: unidimensional and multidimensional. A unidimensional tool will only measure one aspect of the pain, e.g. intensity. Ideally, a multidimensional tool should be used to assess the intricacies of the chronic pain problem. Obviously time is an issue on a busy ward and realistically a quick and simple tool that is comprehensive is unlikely to be found. Therefore, using combinations of different tools is a better compromise. It may be best to use an extensive assessment tool on admission to gain the best possible overview of the problem. Use this assessment to identify the aspect of the problem that concerns the patient the most (usually pain intensity, but maybe lack of sleep or a decline in mood) and measure that aspect of the pain on subsequent assessments. To help identify which may be useful in your clinical area, the following overview will be helpful.

Visual analogue scale (VAS)

This tool consists of a 10 cm line with the markers 'No Pain' on the left hand side of the line and 'Worst Possible Pain' on the right hand side. For example:

No Pain ——————————————————— Worst Possible Pain

The patient is asked where on the line their pain is best represented and to mark the line accordingly. Most patients have no problem with this and are able to fill in the scale. The scale only assesses one dimension of the pain experience, intensity and would therefore not be the scale of choice for extensive assessment. This scale may be more appropriate to gauge the efficacy of a pain relieving action, such as the application of heat or an ice pack. The score is calculated by measuring along the line with a ruler to the patient's mark and the measurement noted. For example, a mark at 78 mm would be scored as 78/100. Small improvements may be identified, which may be helpful in chronic pain states that have been resistant to previous interventions, or when small improvements have been difficult for the patient to identify.

Verbal descriptor scale (VDS)

A verbal descriptor scale also assesses pain intensity. This scale usually consists of three or five numerically graded words. These range, for example, from none to mild to moderate to severe to excruciating, and use a scale of 1 to 5 (or 1 to 3, depending on the number of words) to score the patient's level of pain. Again, this is quick and easy to use. Difficulties with language may be encountered if using a descriptor based scale with a patient who has little understanding of English. It would not be suitable alone as initial assessment, but would indicate improvement or decline after a pain relieving nursing intervention.

Body charts

This tool consists of line drawings of the human form (see Figure 2.1). Front, back and side views can be shown, as well as individual parts of the body, i.e., the feet or the face. This body chart is used to describe location and also extent of pain, i.e., whole arm or whole leg. Also different pains can be identified. This is a common problem when evaluating chronic pain. For example, a patient may be admitted with low back pain. He or she may also complain of bilateral leg pain, reaching the toes on the left and the knee on the right. A relatively new pain being experienced is an ache between the shoulder blades. All these individual pains can be identified on a body chart. Different sites of pain can be labelled for ease of documentation: A = back pain, B = right leg pain, C = etc. The patient may be able to use colours for different areas or even to highlight intensity, although this may become too time-consuming to use at each assessment point; it may be more appropriate as part of the initial assessment in identifying certain aspects of the patient's pain.

Numerical rating scale (NRS)

This scale consists of numerical indicators to show the severity or intensity of the patient's pain. These tools commonly use a 0 to 5 scale (or 0 to 10). The patient is asked to rate their pain on the scale: 0 shows no pain and the numbers increase up the scale to the highest level of pain. This type of scale has several advantages. It is very quick and easy to use, for the patient and the nurse. There is good consistency in interpretation and communication. It is simple to record and is not open to misunderstanding, as a verbal description of pain could be. It can be

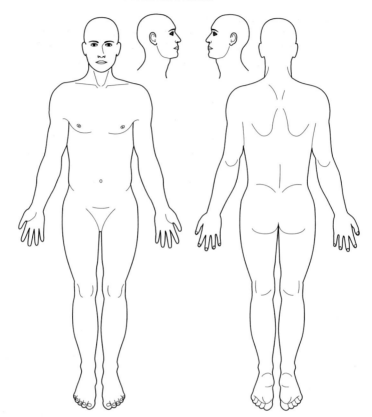

Figure 2.1 Body chart diagram

administered to the patient either in the written form or verbally:

> 'On a scale of 0 to 10, with 0 indicating no pain and 10 being the worse pain you can imagine, can you tell me the number that best describes your pain?'

In the written form, with only minor changes, this scale is simple to explain to non-English speaking patients, or with family or friends acting as interpreters. It can be used to assess the effect of a nursing intervention, but will only record the pain intensity.

The Brief Pain Questionnaire (BPQ)

This tool uses the simplicity of the 0 to 10 intensity scale but applies it to different questions relating to the whole pain experience (see Figure 2.2). It was originally developed for use in cancer care and has been validated in other conditions, such as arthritis.[3] The numerical rating scale has previously been described as straightforward to use. With minimal language changes for patients whose first language is not English, it is still fairly simple to complete. Little explanation is needed to help the patient fill in the form unaided. If the patient is unable to do this, the tool takes only a few minutes for the nurse to describe the area of enquiry for each question.

Previously it has been mentioned that the numerical rating scale will only assess pain intensity, but the 0 to 10 scale of the Brief Pain Questionnaire can be applied to any aspect of the patient's condition. For example, if sleep is a particular problem, the scale can be used each morning, the patient's response noted and intervention can be measured for efficacy. For this reason, the BPQ may be suitable for use on admission. The questionnaire also gives rapid indication of pain relief or

1. Please rate your pain by circling the one number that best describes your pain at its
   worst in the last week:
   0   1   2   3   4   5   6   7   8   9   10
   NO PAIN   WORST PAIN EVER

2. Please rate your pain by circling the one number that best describes your pain on the
   average:
   0   1   2   3   4   5   6   7   8   9   10
   NO PAIN   WORST PAIN EVER

3. Circle the one number that describes how, during the past week, pain has interfered
   with your:

GENERAL ACTIVITY
0   1   2   3   4   5   6   7   8   9   10
DOES NOT INTERFERE   COMPLETELY INTERFERES

MOOD
0   1   2   3   4   5   6   7   8   9   10
DOES NOT INTERFERE   COMPLETELY INTERFERES

WALKING ABILITY
0   1   2   3   4   5   6   7   8   9   10
DOES NOT INTERFERE   COMPLETELY INTERFERES

NORMAL WORK (includes both work outside the home, housework and hobbies)
0   1   2   3   4   5   6   7   8   9   10
DOES NOT INTERFERE   COMPLETELY INTERFERES

RELATIONS WITH OTHER PEOPLE
0   1   2   3   4   5   6   7   8   9   10
DOES NOT INTERFERE   COMPLETELY INTERFERES

SLEEP
0   1   2   3   4   5   6   7   8   9   10
DOES NOT INTERFERE   COMPLETELY INTERFERES

ENJOYMENT OF LIFE
0   1   2   3   4   5   6   7   8   9   10
DOES NOT INTERFERE   COMPLETELY INTERFERES

Figure 2.2 Brief Pain Questionnaire patient assessment form. (From Daut et al., 1983[4] with permission)

deterioration on successive enquiries. The nurse simply asks the patient what number best describes their pain at present, if 0 means no pain and 10 means pain as bad as they can imagine. There is no need to complete further paperwork, the figure given by the patient being recorded as 'Pain Score' on the patient's observation chart, or wherever is convenient for that clinical area.

The Short Form McGill Pain Questionnaire (SFMPQ)

Many of the tools developed to assess and evaluate chronic pain have been developed as research tools. This is to say that while they may be well validated for use in clinical trials and research projects, they may not be suitable for day to day use on a busy acute ward.

The McGill Pain Questionnaire is probably the best example of this point. The MPQ is regarded as the gold standard for chronic pain assessment and has been well validated in many trials. However, the questionnaire is long and complicated to complete. The short form version is quicker to use, but the completion time may still vary enormously depending on the patient (Figure 2.3).

The scale asks the patient to use fifteen descriptive words to describe the pain. The tool also contains a visual analogue scale (VAS) and a present pain intensity (PPI) scale. The patient achieves a score by rating each descriptor as either:

- none (0)
- mild (1)
- moderate (2)
- severe (3)

The patient chooses the descriptor (e.g. cramping) and the corresponding level of intensity at which they feel the pain. This questionnaire is fairly quick to administer once the patient understands what is required – a good explanation is necessary. A patient admitted to a ward in an exacerbation of their chronic pain may be unlikely to grasp the intricacies of the form. One of the problems we have encountered in our Pain Clinic is that patients frequently describe more than one pain (for example back and bilateral leg pain), so which one do they concentrate on to describe? Pain is a very difficult entity to account for: some patients have difficulty describing their pain in this way, or are unable to differentiate between descriptors (e.g. 'gnawing' and 'aching', or 'sharp' and 'stabbing').

In a Chronic Pain Clinic time is specially allocated so that a lengthy pain assessment can take place as part of the patient's usual nursing care. In a ward environment, this period of time is impossible to find, given nurses' numerous other tasks. This scale has been translated into many languages as it is well known in pain research and is referred to in many journal papers. This does not necessarily transfer well to clinical assessment. The MPQ, even in its short form, takes time to administer and may not be entirely practical because of this. It may be appropriate to administer as a baseline, but by definition a baseline implies that

Please indicate the type and severity of your present pain by ticking the appropriate box.

TYPE	NONE	MILD	MODERATE	SEVERE
Throbbing				
Shooting				
Stabbing				
Sharp				
Cramping				
Gnawing				
Hot–Burning				
Aching				
Heavy				
Tender				
Splitting				
Tiring–Exhausting				
Sickening				
Fearful				
Punishing–Cruel				

Please indicate the severity of your pain at present by putting a cross on the line below.

No Pain . . . . Worst Possible Pain

Please indicate the severity of your pain at present by ticking the appropriate box.

No Pain	
Mild	
Discomforting	
Distressing	
Horrible	
Excruciating	

Figure 2.3 The Short Form McGill Pain Questionnaire

further assessments using the same tool will be completed. This is probably not required for a patient on an acute ward. An assessment tool should assess the patient's pain and with repeated administration swiftly show the efficacy of an intervention. The McGill would do this, but not swiftly. The nurse has to fill in a lengthy assessment tool each time, with the patient needing the ability to differentiate between different descriptors and their intensity. Analysing the new information each time would add to this already lengthy process. In this situation the VAS and PPI components of the MPQ will possibly be of more use than filling in the whole form every time. It may be more appropriate to just use a tool that will specify the intensity of the pain compared to the baseline and/or the previous assessment.

More importantly for ward nurses is the actual knowledge that the McGill Pain Questionnaire exists. What it is and how and why it was developed is useful information for nurses involved in pain management. Used correctly, the tool can identify causes of pain and may therefore aid diagnosis. To know that nerve damage pain is often described as burning and neuralgic pains are described by many patients as shooting would be useful in the assessment of the patient's pain.[4]

The Initial Pain Assessment Tool

This tool[5] is designed to be used on admission as the first enquiry about the patient's condition (see Figure 2.4). It is comprehensive and easy to adapt to different clinical areas. It is straightforward to use and fairly self-explanatory. It includes all the areas of importance that are vital to good and complete pain assessment.

1 **Location**. With the aid of the body chart, as described previously, the patient can rapidly show the nurse where the pain is.
2 **Intensity**. This tool allows the assessing nurse the flexibility to decide which method to use when assessing intensity of pain. This is useful as it may vary between patients. Intensity indicators include the verbal descriptor scale, numerical scale or a visual analogue scale. With the VAS it may be best to have blank scales ready to complete on the reverse of the Initial Assessment Tool. Also, space is given so that the intensity tool can be clearly identified, allowing clarity and continuity between different nursing staff.
3 **Quality**. Ask the patient to describe the pain. This is very difficult for many patients. A list of descriptors (such as those from the McGill Pain Questionnaire) may be helpful. Examples include: sharp, gnawing, aching and tiring.
4 **Onset, variations, rhythms**. In this section the nurse will be able to identify factors such as when the pain is worse and what, if anything, improves the pain or makes it worse.
5 **Manner of expressing pain**. The nurse observes the patient and notes non-verbal expressions of pain, body language and verbalization of pain.
6 **What relieves the pain?** It may be helpful to know what the patient does at home or in certain situations to relieve pain. Previous therapies and drugs can be discussed as well. For example, the patient may tell you that the last time he had physiotherapy, a TENS machine was beneficial, but it was only available for a short period of time. Discussion with the ward physiotherapist would be appropriate in this case and a further trial of TENS indicated.

INITIAL PAIN ASSESSMENT TOOL

Date _____

Patient's name _____   Age _____   Ward _____

Diagnosis _____   Doctor _____

Nurse _____

I. LOCATION: Patient or nurse mark drawing:

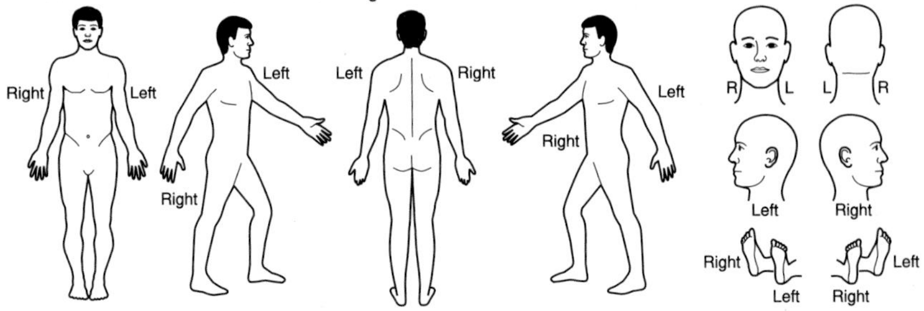

II.   INTENSITY: Patient rates the pain. Scale used:_____

Present: _____

Worse pain gets: _____

Best pain gets: _____

Acceptable level of pain: _____

III.   QUALITY: (use patient's own words, e.g. prick, ache, burn, throb, pull, sharp)_____

IV.   ONSET, DURATION VARIATIONS, RHYTHMS:_____

V.   MANNER OF EXPRESSING PAIN: _____

VI.   WHAT RELIEVES THE PAIN?_____

VII.   WHAT CAUSES OR INCREASES THE PAIN?_____

VIII. EFFECTS OF PAIN: (Note decreased function, decreased quality of life.)

Accompanying symptoms (e.g. nausea) _____

Sleep _____

Appetite _____

Physical activity _____

Relationship with others (e.g. irritability) _____

Emotions (e.g. anger, suicidal, crying) _____

Concentration _____

Other _____

IX.   OTHER COMMENTS: _____

X.   PLAN: _____

Figure 2.4 Initial Pain Assessment Tool. (From McCaffery and Beebe, 1994[5] by permission of Mosby Inc.)

7 **What causes or increases the pain?** This will be important to identify for certain scenarios involving procedures, investigations and general nursing care. The patient tells you that lying flat exacerbates her pain. You know that she is being sent for an MRI scan of the lumbar spine

CONTINUOUS ASSESSMENT SHEET FOR PAIN

Patient _____ Date _____

*Pain rating scale used _____

Purpose: To evaluate the safety and effectiveness of the analgesic(s).
Analgesic(s) prescribed: _____

Time	Pain rating	Analgesic	R	P	BP	Level of arousal	Other[†]	Plan and comments

* *Pain rating:* A number of different scales may be used. Indicate which scale is used and use the same one each time. For example, 0–10 (0 = no pain, 10 = worst pain).
† *Possibilities for other columns:* bowel function, activities, nausea and vomiting, other pain-relief measures. Identify the side effects of greatest concern to patient, family, doctor, nurses.

Figure 2.5 Continuous Assessment Sheet. (From McCaffery and Beebe, 1994[5] by permission of Mosby Inc.)

that involves lying flat for up to 40 minutes or longer. Analgesia can be offered along with an explanation about the scan; the patient will have received improved care. Without good assessment this information may not have been available.

8 **Effects of the pain**. Asking how the pain affects the patient gives a wealth of information. The effects may be physical, psychological, social or financial. Sleep has an important restorative effect and improves the ability to cope: Is the patient able to sleep well or not?

9 **Other comments**. This space is useful to note any miscellaneous detail that the patient or nurse feels important.

10 **Plan**. This is used to outline the specific plan of care for this patient. Recommended times can be recorded here.

Ongoing assessment is recorded on the Continuous Assessment Sheet (Figure 2.5). This sheet can be amended to show 'Intervention' or 'Analgesia', whichever is most appropriate for that ward area. Other columns may be included such as bowel function, activities or nausea/vomiting depending on the patient's general medical condition.

Implementing change in busy, acute ward areas is notoriously difficult. The reasons for introduction of a new (or to replace an existing) pain assessment tool must be relevant and identified as a real need. Otherwise, human nature and the present escalating workload of the nursing staff will combine to quash any innovations that are to be introduced. A simple patient satisfaction questionnaire may be helpful in identifying areas of care that could be improved upon. If pain is raised as an issue by the patients, then that issue becomes hard to ignore. With this in mind, action can then be taken to improve the patients' pain relief whilst they are inpatients on the ward. In order to achieve this, skilful assessment is the key to improving pain control. If you decide to implement a new assessment form for monitoring pain levels, communication is absolutely vital at all levels and on every shift. Many staff meetings will be needed and a trial period should be agreed. If after six months the original patient satisfaction questionnaire is repeated, improvements may be shown.

The patient with chronic pain presents an immense challenge to nursing care because the patient may well be wary about the intentions and beliefs of the nursing staff. These counter-productive feelings will be based on their experiences of previous contact with the health services, which can be highly negative. In particular the enquiries that the nurse is required to make about the patient's condition during pain assessment may go some way to influencing the whole outcome of the admission. The challenge for the nurse lies in the ability to empathize, listen and re-educate. These are the mainstays of chronic pain nursing.

Summary
- Patients have all the information required for assessment – listen to them.
- Believe the patient – it is essential to establish trust in the nurse/patient relationship.
- Identify the potential problem of bias – assimilate the information received without judging the patient.
- Recognize that the patient's expectations can vary tremendously from those of the nurse.
- Exclude bias and varying interpretations by using a simple pain assessment tool.
- Assessment establishes a purposeful route of communication, which may positively influence the patient's outcome.

References

1. International Association for the Study of Pain Sub Committee on Taxonomy (1979) Pain terms: a list with definitions and notes on usage. *Pain*, 6, 249–52.
2. McCaffrey, M. (1979) *Nursing the Patient in Pain.* New York: Harper and Row.
3. Melzack, R. (1987) The Short Form McGill Pain Questionnaire. *Pain*, 30, 191–7.
4. Daut, R. L., Cleeland, C. S. and Flanery, R. C. (1983) Development of the Brief Pain Questionnaire to Assess Pain in Cancer and other diseases. *Pain*, 17, 197–210.
5. McCaffery, M. and Beebe, A. (1994) *Pain: Clinical Manual for Nursing Practice* (UK edition). London: Mosby.

Pain syndromes

J. F. Hazelgrove and C. Price

Definitions

The definition of pain offered by the International Association for the Study of Pain is as follows:

> An unpleasant sensory and emotional experience associated with actual or potential tissue damage, or described in terms of such damage.[1]

This states explicitly that pain always has a subjective component. It is both a physiological sensation and an emotional reaction to that sensation.

There are several pain syndromes that are seen in the Pain Clinic. The diagnosis and management of these syndromes frequently requires a multidisciplinary approach. The effects of chronic pain are physical (inability to perform daily tasks or work) and psychological (depression, isolation and loss of self-esteem). Thus, both aspects must be addressed in order to treat an individual successfully.

Types of pain

There are two types of pain: **nociceptive** and **neuropathic**.

- Nociceptive pain can be divided into somatic and visceral, and is triggered by pain sensors that sense mechanical stimulation, heat and touch. The pain tends to be of the acute type and is appropriate.
- Neuropathic pain occurs when a nerve is injured or sends faulty messages. It carries on for a long time after the initial stimulus and is inappropriate. The processes involved in neuropathic pain are not fully understood but abnormal sensitization is involved.

Nociceptors

Nociceptors are neurological receptors capable of differentiating between innocuous and noxious stimuli. They are the undifferentiated terminals of Aδ and C fibres, which are the thinnest myelinated and unmyelinated fibres respectively. Aδ fibres are also called high-threshold mechano-receptors. They respond primarily to mechanical stimuli of noxious intensity.

Common terms used to describe pain sensation

Allodynia

A non-noxious stimulus causes pain, e.g. stroking or moving a joint. Common in many neuropathic pain syndromes, e.g. post-herpetic neuralgia, complex regional pain syndrome (CRPS).

Allogenic substances

Substances released from injured tissues (or which are injected) cause sensitization or activation of nociceptors.

Anaesthesia dolorosa

Pain occurs in an area that is otherwise numb or desensitized. For example, patients with trigeminal neuralgia are sometimes treated with radiofrequency lesioning of the trigeminal nerve. They may go on to experience pain in a now denervated area.

Analgesia

The opposite – a noxious stimulus causes no pain.

Dysaesthesia

A painful paraesthesia, e.g. 'burning feet' felt in alcoholic peripheral neuropathy.

Hyperpathia

An abnormally intense painful response to repetitive stimuli; that is, too much pain. Usually a single stimulus is not painful although multiple stimuli are (summation dysaesthesia). This is a feature of neuropathic pain.

Hypoaesthesia

Decreased sensitivity to stimulation (local anaesthesia).

Neuralgia

Pain in the distribution of a nerve or nerves. It is often characteristic, being electrical, shock-like pain, e.g. trigeminal neuralgia.

Table 3.1 Common pain conditions seen in Pain Clinics

Pain syndrome	Examples
Non-specific musculoskeletal pain	Low back pain, neck pain, fibromyalgia
Neuropathic pain	Phantom limb pain, CRPS, diabetic neuropathy, central post-stroke pain
Headache, facial pain	Trigeminal neuralgia, atypical facial pain
Inflammatory disease	Rheumatoid arthritis
Visceral pain	Chronic pancreatitis
Genitourinary pain	Pelvic pain, testicular pain
Neoplastic disease refractory to standard analgesia	Chest wall pain, nerve root invasion

Source: Merskey, H. and Bogduk, N. (1994)[1]

Paraesthesia

Any abnormal sensation. It may be spontaneous or evoked, e.g. 'pins and needles' pain associated with sciatica.

Table 3.1 shows a classification of common pain syndromes.

Musculoskeletal pain

Low back pain

Low back pain accounts for between 26 and 50% of referrals to a pain unit.[2] Low back pain affects 80% of the population at some point in their lives and the incidence is increasing. It also accounts for 120 million working days lost per annum. There is a high socio-economic cost as it affects the working population to such an extent that they often have to cease working or take up less demanding jobs.

Low back problems often occur following a minor injury in poorly conditioned, unfit people. The resulting increased lordosis, combined with pre-existing poor abdominal muscle tone, means that weight bearing is shifted to the posterior structure. There is maximal loading on the facet joints, shear forces on the discs and compression of the intervertebral foramina. The problems that result are disc herniation, facet joint pain, single nerve root pain and myofascial pain. Degenerative disease produces similar problems. It is important to exclude serious systemic disease. This has usually been done by the time the patient reaches a pain clinic.

As the problem is multifaceted, treatment often requires a multi-disciplinary approach;[3] this should include physiotherapy, a review of medications and some alternative pain relief in order to facilitate physio-therapy. This may include transcutaneous nerve stimulation (TENS) and injection therapy. Physiotherapy should exercise and stretch stiff joints, support structures and muscles and restore abdominal tone. General exercises in the form of a graded exercise programme can also be helpful in improving overall level of fitness.

It is difficult to separate the causes of back pain into component parts, yet this is often done in order to facilitate treatment. The term posterior compartment syndrome may be more appropriate. Equally, imaging is often unhelpful in the diagnosis of these problems. A classification into these parts is as follows.

Facet syndrome

This may present as dull, aching, low back pain radiating to the buttocks and thigh (although the pain may radiate anywhere). Extension worsens the pain. There is tenderness over facet joints. Tendon reflexes and straight leg raising may be diminished. Diagnosis is usually by diagnostic facet joint blockade, although the use of these has been questioned. Facet joint pain may accompany spinal stenosis and degenerative joint disease. The aim of physiotherapy is to strengthen surrounding structures and reduce loading on those structures.

Acute disc syndromes

Here pain is sharp and radiates in the distribution of the nerve. Pain is better on lying down and worse on coughing and straining. Straight leg raising is diminished and there is often muscle spasm. The pain may often be accompanied by low back pain. Other problems may occur concurrently such as facet joint syndrome and spinal stenosis. Treatment may consist of an epidural steroid injection to help root pain (although these are short-acting only), gentle physiotherapy stretches and regular analgesia.

Failed back syndrome (FBS)

This is back pain or associated pain that recurs after back surgery.[4] It presents usually as low back pain with sharp, often burning pain radiating to the thighs, buttocks or calf. It is often difficult to differentiate between previous signs that occurred before surgery and new signs. FBS may occur because of inadequate patient selection, inadequate surgery, the wrong diagnosis (many have spinal stenosis), fibrosis and scarring or co-incidental pathology.

Treatment should, in the first instance, aim to provide symptomatic relief and restore function; many will require psychological support to deal with the failure and persistent pain. Direct spinal cord stimulation is thought to help. This involves insertion of an electrode into the epidural space, with stimulation being controlled by the patient. This tends to help the radicular pain, but not the back pain. The potential complications of this technique should be borne in mind. Frequently, a multidisciplinary pain management programme is necessary.[5]

Myofascial pain

Here multiple trigger points predominate. Myofascial pain may occur anywhere in the body but is most commonly found in the back (lumbar or cervical). Gentle stretch combined with relaxation may reduce spasm. Trigger point injections may provide short-term relief.

Piriformis syndrome

This may present in a similar fashion to sciatica due to prolapsed disc. However, low back pain does not usually occur with piriformis syndrome and radicular symptoms predominate, worsening over the day. A prominent buttock with many trigger points is present. Treatment options may include stretch and relaxation of the affected muscle, surgery or botulinum toxin.

Sacro-iliac joint dysfunction

Here, the pain is dull, aching and radiating to the thigh. It is worse when lifting and sitting. There may be low back spasm. Treatment is directed towards improved mobility and analgesia. TENS is often helpful, as is sacro-iliac joint injection.

Spinal stenosis

This is pain that occurs possibly because the blood supply is restricted to the spinal cord, usually because of arthritis. The pain comes on when walking and gets better by leaning forward or sitting down. Epidurals or surgery can often be effective treatments. However, the sufferer is often elderly and frail, limiting the treatment options.

A summary of therapies and their application in low back pain is shown in Table 3.2.

Neck pain

Approximately 9% of men and 12% of women will have neck complaints.[6] The annual new episode incidence rate per 1000 person-years is 12.1 in soft tissue rheumatic neck disorders in primary care cases attending medical services.[7] Motor vehicle accidents account for a sizeable portion of neck complaints, with 24% of subjects experiencing persistent symptoms at 12 months post injury.[8] The main problems that are seen are cervical spondylosis and whiplash syndrome.

Cervical spondylosis

In this condition the nerve roots in the neck are being compressed either by arthritic joints or cartilage. Pain is usually generalized, although it can be localized to one nerve root. It may be distributed to the face or anterior chest wall, and a headache can occur (usually occipito-frontal). There

Table 3.2 Summary of treatments for chronic low back pain and evaluation of effectiveness

Therapies	Manual treatments	Neuromodulation	Injection therapy	Medications	Pain management programme	Surgery
Examples	**Physiotherapy** Back School not effective Operant procedures coupled with physical reconditioning effective	**TENS** Not effective in the long term	**Trigger points** Not helpful	**NSAIDs** Not generally helpful	**Physiotherapy** Graded exercise programme	**Discectomy** Microdiscectomy may be more useful Little data
	Chiropractic	**Spinal cord stimulation** May be effective for FBS	**Intra-articular facet joint injections** Possibly short-term gains	**Paracetamol** Minimal help	**Occupational therapy** Goal-setting and pacing	**Discolysis** No strong evidence for use
	Osteopathy		**Denervation**	**Opioids** Side-effects outweigh the benefits	**Psychology** Cognitive-behavioural interventions	**Fusion** Instability
			Epidural steroid injection Short-term gain	**Anti-depressants**	**Medication management**	
					Relaxation Operant component	
Comments	Little evidence comparing manual therapies to standard physiotherapy		Majority short-term gains		A combination of these is highly effective long term	

Source: Evans, G. and Richards, S. (1996)[3]

may be sensory disturbances in the dermatomes related to that nerve while reduced reflexes and wasting in corresponding muscles may occur. Cervical myelopathy may be seen if the spinal cord is compressed, causing weakness in the lower limbs and nerve root pain in the upper limbs. Vertigo, visual disturbances and vertebrobasilar insufficiency, if present, may result in dizziness and nausea.

Referral to a neurosurgeon is necessary if this presents acutely. Cervical epidural injection may provide short-term pain relief.

Whiplash syndrome[9]

Whiplash occurs either as a result of car or sports injury when the neck is bent very quickly, damaging the ligaments and other soft tissues. There may also be bony injury, with damage to the discs and small neck joints. Those who are not better within 3 months are unlikely to get better, thereby developing chronic neck pain. The usual pain is dull and aching in the upper neck and occiput. Headache often develops, again at the back of the head. Tingling and numbness in the hands especially the ring and little finger are common. Sympathetic dysfunction, dizziness and visual disturbances may also occur. Treatment mainstay is physiotherapy and analgesia. It is important to keep the neck mobile. Cervical facet joint injections have been reported to be of some benefit, and anecdotally TENS is useful.

Neuropathic pain

Neuropathic pain differs considerably from nociceptive pain. Rather than being sharp and localized the pain is diffuse and burning in character. Areas of allodynia and hyperalgesia are usually found. Neuropathic pain can be particularly difficult to treat. Conventional analgesics often fail to work. Therefore, patients have often been through a variety of treatments, have high levels of distress and abnormal beliefs. This must also be managed psychologically, in addition to providing pain relief, if treatment is to be effective.

Common neuropathic pain problems are shown in Table 3.3.

Complex regional pain syndromes (CRPS)

Complex regional pain syndromes are chronically painful conditions usually involving the limbs, and are characterized by burning pain, loss of function and skin changes. There are two types of regional pain syndromes, one that affects the whole of a distal part of a limb (CRPS I) and one that occurs in the distribution of a nerve (CRPS II). The pain usually follows trauma and is subsequent on disuse of that limb. The patient complains of allodynia and hyperalgesia. The limb often appears pale, swollen and shiny and there may be a temperature difference from the unaffected limb. The patient becomes afraid to use the limb because of the pain, which then worsens the situation.

Table 3.3 Common neuropathic pain conditions

Trigeminal neuralgia

Post-herpetic neuralgia

Scar pain
  —inguinal herniorrhaphy
  —hysterectomy
  —thoracotomy

Phantom limb pain

Complex regional pain syndromes

Central post-stroke pain

Neuropathies
  —diabetic
  —alcoholic
  —ischaemic
  —irradiation
  —chemotherapy

Treatment is aimed at encouraging use of that limb whilst prescribing analgesia. Effective analgesia can often be achieved with TENS, sympathetic blocks such as stellate ganglion blockade, and adjuvant analgesics such as amitriptyline and anticonvulsants. The use of sympathetic blocks is controversial. If successful pain relief is achieved with intravenous phentolamine then this suggests that it may respond to sympathetic blockade. Guanethidine blocks have been used for many years, but their effect may be more related to compression or ischaemia rather than to the drug itself.

Maintenance of mobility is fundamental to the recovery from this condition. The patient becomes afraid to use the limb because of the pain, the situation worsens and a vicious cycle is established. Behavioural management may ultimately be necessary if other interventions fail.

Post-herpetic neuralgia (PHN)

PHN occurs after an acute outbreak of herpes zoster. Pain is often described as gnawing, with paroxysmal shooting or shocking pains. Very light stimulation can trigger the pain. There may be pigmentation scarring over the areas of hyperaesthesia and allodynia. Lesions are in the dorsal nerve root. The elderly and immunosuppressed are commonly those affected.

This condition can be very difficult to treat. Early use of aciclovir or steroids may reduce the risk of it occurring. Treatment is with tricyclic antidepressants (e.g. amitriptyline), in the first instance. In the more resistant cases capsaicin cream may be of benefit although this may be painful to apply. Anticonvulsants such as carbamazepine, lamotrigine and more recently gabapentin may help. The usefulness of these drugs, particularly in the elderly, is limited by their side-effect profile. Although nerve blocks have been used quite extensively in the past there is no evidence to support their use.

Diabetic neuropathic pain

Diabetic neuropathy is the commonest example of a metabolic disorder causing neuropathic pain (up to 7.5% patients seen in a Diabetic Clinic complain of neuropathic pain[10]). The small nerve endings get damaged over time due to the effects of raised glucose itself. However, the precise mechanism causing the pain is still a matter for discussion. In addition, joint disease and vascular disease may cause pain. The pain is described as burning, tingling or shooting. Treatment is by maintaining use of the affected limb, antidepressants, capsaicin, TENS and anticonvulsants. Sympathetic blocks may sometimes be effective.

Phantom limb pain

Patients may experience phantom sensation, phantom pain and/or stump pain. These are not synonymous terms. Phantom sensation refers to non-painful sensations only, compared with phantom pain, which refers to painful sensations. Stump pain refers to pain at the site of an amputation. Any amputated limb, appendage or viscera can be affected, including teeth. Most published research refers to the treatment of phantom limb pain. Once established, phantom pain can consume a patient's quality of life.

It is unclear whether the same physiological mechanisms are responsible for each symptom type; the frequency with which they are seen varies.

The incidence of phantom pain may be as high as 95% in amputees. The size of the problem is difficult to ascertain. There is probably under-reporting due to reluctance amongst this usually older age group to admit that they have phantom phenomena and, until recent years, many physicians presumed this condition to be 'in the mind'.

Following limb amputation, patients usually describe sensation in the distal part of the missing limb. The size of the limb may telescope down in size over time. They may describe painful distortions of the missing hand/foot, though more often burning, crushing or lancinating pain occurs. It can be influenced or triggered by external or internal factors, including the weather and emotions.

Phantom pain can take months to appear and can even increase in severity in 5–10% of patients. More commonly it arises soon after amputation and attacks resolve or diminish within one to two years. The condition is not static and changes character over the first year. There is an early pain which can occur a few days postoperatively, and a chronic pain which can develop from the initial pain or present for the first time several years later. There is often a similarity between preoperative pain and phantom pain.

Prevention of the condition is felt to be better than attempting cures later. There is evidence to suggest that noxious stimuli can generate permanent long-term changes within the central nervous system. Thus, pre-emptive analgesia has been attempted using preoperative epidural analgesia, in order to reduce pain before amputation. This is usually inserted the day before surgery as the decision to amputate is often only made at this late stage. Therefore, alternative methods of pain relief would seem a more practical alternative. Other centres concentrate on reducing intraoperative and postoperative pain by other means. A catheter can be placed alongside cut nerves during surgery and local anaesthetic infused from that point for several days postoperatively. This is referred to as continual postoperative regional analgesia.

Reviewing the literature does not provide any evidence of long-term benefit using either technique, in terms of the reduction in the rate of phantom pain by one year after amputation. Epidural analgesia is not without risk. It is impossible to comment on whether insertion of an epidural one week before surgery would affect long-term outcome, but in reality this would never be practicable and usually not possible.

An almost endless list of drugs has been used to treat phantom phenomena; many have met with some success. They have been tried as a result of perceived benefits in other types of neuropathic pain. Conventional analgesics such as NSAIDs and opiates are usually not considered appropriate for neuropathic pain. There is no evidence-based rationale for their use in phantom pain. There are, however, numerous anecdotal case reports of benefits for those patients using these drugs, and it is generally felt that they have a role to play in some cases. Intrathecal buprenorphine may produce very good results in some patients.

There is some evidence that a calcitonin infusion may reduce phantom pain postoperatively, and prevent its recurrence over time. Ketamine has also been used with some good effects. The problem with both calcitonin and ketamine is the emergence of adverse side-effects, limiting their usage. Mixing ketamine with benzodiazepines or droperidol may reduce the incidence of side-effects.

There is good evidence for the efficacy of carbamazepine in trigeminal neuralgia; however, there are only a few case reports supporting its use in phantom pain. Clonazepam has been successfully used to treat lancinating phantom pain. The role of gabapentin is unclear.

Phantom pain appears to affect most amputees at some stage. Sadly, many chronic sufferers have been unable to find relief for their symptoms. It seems no single treatment will benefit large numbers of sufferers, but there are over sixty reported treatments which have had excellent results for some. TENS and physiotherapy undoubtedly can be very useful, especially in stump pain.

Medical and surgical advances should aim to reduce the number of amputations performed; thereafter, a multidisciplinary approach is required. Patient education is important in alleviating stress associated with phantom pain, and suggesting coping strategies is helpful. Pain management programmes may be useful. Future research must be directed towards prevention, but for those patients already suffering new therapies may arise such as new NMDA antagonists, cyclooxygenase inhibitors and the cannabinoids.

A summary of therapies is shown in Table 3.4.

Headache and facial pain

Headache

Headache is the most common reason for attendance with pain at a general practice, although it does not have the social costs of low back pain, as it tends to be less disabling. There are many causes of headache, and the majority of patients are referred to a neurology clinic. Most chronic headache syndromes can be identified by conducting a careful interview to yield a thorough understanding of the patient's headache. The interview should explore the 'PQRST' of the pain: Provocation, Quality, Region, Strength and Time course, with the last element being the most helpful.[11] A list of all current medicines, and their frequency of use, should be obtained, since the overuse of various analgesics can convert paroxysmal migraine into chronic daily headache. Psychosocial issues should be addressed, since depression can manifest as chronic headache. During examination, any focal findings warrant tomographic imaging of the brain. Findings on physical examination, however, are usually normal in patients with chronic headache.

There are three common presentations to a pain clinic:

- tension headache
- cervicogenic headache
- myofascial pain giving rise to headache (see above)

Tension headache

Tension headache is extremely common, and onset is often gradual; usually neck pain is involved. It presents as a band-like, bilateral pulsatile ache. It is of gradual onset lasting several days. Sleep disturbance is common. Stress is a common trigger. Pre-existing conditions of spondylitis and whiplash may exacerbate it.

Treatment is dependent on patient factors. If it occurs only occasionally then relaxation techniques, non-steroidal drugs and education about avoiding risk factors may be all that is needed. If it is intractable then antidepressants, non-steroidals and paracetamol should be considered. However, analgesia must be prescribed with care as their use often leads to rebound headache. This is especially the case with paracetamol.

Chronic daily headache is defined as headaches occurring at least 5 days per week for at least 1 year. They are associated with nausea and vomiting. Common aggravating factors include physical activity, bending over, noise, stress or tension, and menstruation.

Table 3.4 Neuropathic pain treatment modalities

Treatment modalities	Treatment	Example	Specific conditions	Comments
Manual therapies	Physiotherapy		CRPS, stump and phantom pain	TENS also helps
Injection therapy	Sympathetic blockade	Stellate ganglion blockade Lumbar sympathectomy Guanethidine blockade	Facial pain CRPS Peripheral vascular disease	
	Nerve block	Genitofemoral block	Post-inguinal herniorrhaphy pain Thoracotomy pain	
	Infiltration	Intercostal nerve block	Post-sternotomy scar pain	
Neuromodulation	Spinal cord stimulation TENS		CRPS, post-cordotomy dysaesthesia CRPS, most neuropathic pain	
Medication	Antidepressants	Amitriptyline	Diabetic neuropathy (DN) Central post-stroke pain Trigeminal neuralgia	
	Anticonvulsants	Carbamazepine, gabapentin Phenytoin	Post-herpetic neuralgia (PHN) Migraine	Often limited by side-effects
	Deplete Substance P	Capsaicin	Phantom pain	
	NMDA antagonists	Ketamine Dextromethorphan	Central pain	

Cervicogenic headache

Cervicogenic headache presents as unilateral headache with prominent involvement of the neck. Common causes are whiplash injury and osteoarthritis of the neck. Pain is provoked by pressure on the ipsilateral neck and there is reduced movement. Pain is usually worse in the morning and is relieved by relaxation. C1 to C3 nerves are involved together with the facet joints of C2/3.

Treatment is aimed at providing sufficient pain relief to get the neck mobile again. Therefore, physiotherapy is the mainstay of treatment. There are several possible therapies: acupuncture and TENS are often effective. Greater occipital nerve blocks and cervical facet joint injections are more invasive methods, with the latter providing longer-term pain relief.

Myofascial pain

See above.

Common headache conditions and their treatments are summarized in Table 3.5.

Facial pain

Patients with facial pain may present to a neurologist, maxillo-facial surgeon or a Pain Clinic. The two most common conditions seen in the Pain Clinic are trigeminal neuralgia and atypical facial pain. Post-herpetic neuralgia affecting the Vth cranial nerve may also be seen.

Trigeminal neuralgia

Trigeminal neuralgia is pain produced in the area of the trigeminal nerve. It is more common in women than in men, in middle age and in patients with multiple sclerosis. It may also occur with tumours invading the trigeminal nerve. In most cases the abnormality is thought to be an abnormal vessel compressing the nerve in the base of the skull.

Pain usually occurs in the mandibular region. It is described as a series of electric shocks, lasting a few seconds only, on one side of the face. This may occur several times a day and can make the patient suicidal. Pain is triggered by light touch. Therefore, washing, shaving and cleaning teeth become very difficult. There is often little to find on examination.

Most patients can be treated with anticonvulsants for long periods of time, usually carbamazepine. If medical management fails then usually surgical treatment is indicated. This involves microvascular decompression or neurectomy of the trigeminal nerve. If patients are frail, suffer from multiple sclerosis, or do not wish to undergo craniotomy then radiofrequency lesioning is usually indicated. This is often highly effective for a few years but the pain tends to recur.

Table 3.5 Headache conditions and their treatments

Condition	Clinical features	Therapy	Comments
Migraine	Aura Unilateral, pulsating, stops activity, worse when doing something, photophobia, tunnel vision, speech disturbed, nausea and vomiting	*Prevention* Avoid triggers, beta-blockers, pizotifen *Treatment* NSAIDs, sumatriptan, paracetamol, relaxation	Most do not have aura
Cervicogenic headache	Headache due to upper cervical nerve roots irritation	Steroid injections to upper facet joints help TENS and physiotherapy	
Tension headache	Pressing, mild, bilateral Not worse with activity No nausea or vomiting	Antidepressants Sumatriptan Relaxation and cognitive strategies	Avoid analgesic overuse as this may cause rebound headache

Atypical facial pain

This is facial pain for which no pathology can be demonstrated. It is described as diffuse, aching without trigger zones. It often occurs in women aged 30–50. Often sufferers have had numerous dental procedures and failed medical procedures. Treatment is therefore focused on pain management rather than palliation of symptoms.

Post-herpetic neuralgia

Although post-herpetic neuralgia can affect any nerve, it often affects the ophthalmic division of the trigeminal nerve and is common in the elderly.

Pain associated with medical conditions

This includes a variety of conditions where chronic pain is a prominent feature of the disease. Frequent flare-ups, the impact on body structures such as bones and joints, and compliance with long-term medication are often the problems. Patients are often very fearful of doing further damage and may fail therefore to achieve their potential mobility. Such conditions include the following.

Rheumatoid arthritis

Neck, shoulder and hip pains are the most common pain problems encountered. Blocks are often very helpful in providing medium-term pain relief.

Diabetes

The usual pain problems are diabetic neuropathy and painful ulcers (see above).

Vascular disease

This may include intractable angina and peripheral vascular disease. Here, sympathetic blocks can be most helpful in palliation of symptoms.

Multiple sclerosis

Long tract neuropathic pain may occur; also, muscle spasms and flare-ups may be extremely painful. Cannabinoids are helpful, although rehabilitation strategies may help in improving quality of life.

Urogenital pain

Pelvic pain

Many women have chronic pelvic pain without any gynaecological abnormality or 'obvious pathology' (CPPWOP). The pain is described as a dull, cramping ache, worse before menstruation. Pelvic examination reveals a diffuse tenderness. It was formerly described as pelvic congestion syndrome. It is thought that altered autonomic activity exists, leading to altered blood flow and pain. Non-steroidal anti-inflammatory drugs and hormone therapy are helpful. Sometimes blockade of the pre-sacral nerves can help but generally psychological input is essential. Although a pain-specific cognitive-behavioural approach can be used, there are often issues about sexuality that are best covered individually by specialist attention.

Laparoscopy has made the diagnosis of pelvic pain more specific, although this does not mean that it is any easier to manage!

Pelvic adhesions

Pelvic adhesions can be entirely unrelated to the degree of pain experienced. Adhesiolysis is not of long-term benefit and the approach should be similar to CPPWOP.

Haematuria–loin syndrome

This is loin pain occurring with blood in the urine with no other abnormality found. Frequently these patients have had many investigations and are taking many drugs. Therefore, a general pain management approach is most helpful, although ureteric injection of capsaicin has been described. This is excruciatingly painful, and an epidural is needed to overcome this. Autotransplantation is also thought to be useful.

Interstitial cystitis

This is cystitis without any organism found to be responsible for the symptoms. Bladder wall abnormalities are found. It is easy to confuse with pelvic pain or irritable bowel syndrome. Ablation of the nerves to the bladder has been reported to provide long-term benefit although, again, pain management may be the best approach.

Testicular pain

Testicular pain commonly occurs after vasectomy. It affects 10% of all cases. Other testicular pains may be due to chronic low grade infection.

Treatment of testicular pain is difficult. Antibiotic therapy such as tetracycline or a quinolone, often combined with a non-steroidal anti-inflammatory drug, may be useful – in some cases even when infection has not been identified. Spermatic cord block and transcutaneous electrical nerve stimulation may help relieve pain, although it often recurs. Antidepressants sometimes relieve the pain. Many patients benefit from a pain management programme. When all conservative efforts have failed and testicular pain continues to diminish the patient's quality of life orchidectomy may have to be considered. In general, surgery should be undertaken only when a pathologic condition is found and not for pain relief alone. Phantom pain may occur after this.[12]

Visceral pain

Visceral pain occurs as a result of activation of pain sensors in the walls of the organs in the abdomen. The pain may be felt within the abdomen or referred elsewhere, e.g. shoulder tip pain from the gallbladder.

The visceral organs do not feel many pain stimuli such as cutting. They do feel distension, traction, twisting and stretch. This means that pain is often poorly localized and the cause may be in a different area from the pain. Pain may be from:

- **epigastrium**, such as duodenal ulcer pain, which is pain that is relieved by eating
- **peri-umbilical region**, when small bowel pain is worse when eating and better fasting
- **lower abdomen**, irritable bowel or pelvic pain may be causes
- **intra-abdominal organs**, e.g. chronic pancreatitis

Abdominal pain that occurs in discrete attacks with gaps in between is more likely to have recognizable pathology than abdominal pain that continues for weeks and is unrelenting.

Many of those with chronic abdominal pain report sexual or physical abuse. This makes management complex. Patients often make some gains from a pain management approach but less so than comparable patients with musculoskeletal disorders. Other treatments that may be helpful include acupuncture, opioids and coeliac plexus blockade.

Cancer pain that is refractory to standard treatment approaches

Cancer pain can usually be treated according to WHO guidelines and judicious use of adjuvant agents by those specializing in palliative care. Approximately 10% of cancer pains will be difficult to treat and may require an invasive approach. This must be done with the emphasis on quality of life. Pain in cancer may occur because of:

- **nociceptive** pain due to tumour invasion of pain-sensitive structures
- **neuropathic** pain due to invasion of a nerve plexus

- **incidental pain**: pain that occurs that is unrelated to the cancer
- pain due to **treatments**[13]

Bone metastases are the most commonly painful cancers. Pain that occurs in movement due to invasion of the moving structure is also very painful, and refractory to oral agents, e.g. chest wall invasion in mesothelioma, pathological fracture of a hip. Pain Clinics tend to provide ablative therapy such as intrathecal neurolysis or cordotomy to relieve pain where other, less invasive, measures have failed. Other therapies that are useful are irradiation of a bony metastasis, and surgical fixation of a pathological fracture and these should also be considered. Psychological issues must be addressed, such as fear of pain and fear of dying. Psychoeducational care has been found to benefit adults with cancer in relation to anxiety and depression.[14] Interventions such as general psychodynamic counselling and cognitive-behavioural counselling, e.g. problem-solving skill development and education, should be considered.

Common conditions seen in the Pain Clinic include the following.

Post-mastectomy pain

This may be due to scar pain, intercostobrachial neuralgia, post-irradiation brachioplexopathy and invasion of the brachial plexus with tumour.

Treatment of the plexus invasion can often be achieved with adjuvant agents such as carbamazepine. Amitriptyline and local infiltration with steroid is useful for scar and arm pain.[15]

Epidural invasion by tumour

Epidural steroid injection is often helpful. TENS can be useful for low back pain.

Epidural clonidine may provide effective relief for intractable cancer pain, particularly of the neuropathic type.[16]

Pancreatic or other visceral pain due to carcinoma

Neurolytic Coeliac Plexus Blockade (NCPB) is likely to have long lasting analgesic efficacy for pancreatic and other types of intra-abdominal cancer. Short-term outcomes show a high rate (86–96%) of successful NCPB regardless of the radiological techniques used. Adverse effects such as hypotension and diarrhoea are common, but transient.[17]

Bony metastases

Neural blockade, intrathecal opioid infusions and adjuvant infusions are often helpful.

Specific procedures

Cordotomy

This may be helpful for unilateral tumours, particularly chest wall invasion and pelvic tumours that are slow growing. Dysaesthesias afterwards may outweigh its usefulness.

Intrathecal neurolysis

This may be helpful for unilateral lower body cancers or perineal tumours. There is a high chance of sacral nerve destruction, leading to incontinence, and this should be considered in the appropriateness of therapy.

Summary
- The mechanisms of chronic pain, despite much effort, are still poorly understood.
- Psychological factors are as important as physical factors in understanding the impact of chronic pain on an individual's life.
- Management should be multidisciplinary. The emphasis should be on improving physical and social functioning, and on management of fluctuating levels of chronic pain.
- The role of many therapies is unclear in the long-term. A cognitive-behavioural approach is one of the most successful treatment options.
- Back pain is the most common chronic pain syndrome, and has an enormous financial and social impact.

References

1. Merskey, H. and Bogduk, N. (eds) (1994) *Classification of Chronic Pain*, 2nd edn. Seattle, WA: IASP Press.
2. McQuay, H. and Moore, A. (1998) *An Evidence Based Source of Pain Relief.* Oxford: Oxford University Press.
3. Evans, G. and Richards, S. (1996) *Low Back Pain: a Review of Therapeutic Interventions.* University of Bristol Health Care Evaluation Unit.
4. Long, D. M. (1991) Failed low back syndrome. *Neurosurgical Clinics of North America*, 2, 899–912.
5. Rocco, A. G., Frank, E., Kaul, A. F., Lipson, S. J. and Gallo, J. P. (1989) Epidural steroids, epidural morphine and epidural steroids combined with morphine in the treatment of post-laminectomy syndrome. *Pain*, 36, 297–303.
6. Lawrence, J. S. (1969) Disc degeneration: its frequency and relationship to symptoms. *Annals of Rheumatological Disease*, 28, 121–37.
7. Royal College of Practitioners (1980) *Third National Morbidity Survey in General Practice.* London: HMSO.
8. Radanov, B. P., Sturzenegger, M., DeStefano, G. and Schindrig, A. (1994) Relationship between early somatic, radiological, cognitive and psychosocial findings and outcome during a one-year follow-up in 117 patients suffering from common whiplash. *British Journal of Rheumatology*, 33, 442–8.
9. Barnsley, L., Lord, S. and Bogduk, N. (1994) Whiplash injury: a review. *Pain*, 58, 283–307.

10. MacFarlane, B. V., Wright, A., O'Callahan, J. and Benson, H. A. C. (1997) Chronic Neuropathic Pain and its control by drugs. *Pharmacological Therapy*, 95, 1–19.
11. Ryan, C.W. (1996) Evaluation of patients with chronic headache. *American Family Physician*, 54(3), 1051–7.
12. Baum, N. and Defidio, L. (1995) Chronic testicular pain: a work-up and treatment guide for the primary care physician. *Postgraduate Medicine*, 98, 151–8.
13. Melzack, R. and Wall, P. D. (1994) *Textbook of Pain*, 3rd edn. Edinburgh: Churchill Livingstone.
14. Devine, E. C. and Westlake, S. K. (1995) The effects of psychoeducational care provided to adults with cancer: meta-analysis of 116 studies. *Oncology Nursing Forum*, 22 (9), 1369–81.
15. The Steering Committee on Clinical Practice Guidelines for the Care and Treatment of Breast Cancer (1998) The management of chronic pain in patients with breast cancer. *Journal of the Canadian Medical Association*, 158 (3), S71–S81.
16. Eisenach, J. C., DuPen, S., Dubois, M., Miguel, R. and Allin, D. (1995) Epidural clonidine analgesia for intractable cancer pain: the Epidural Clonidine Study Group. *Pain*, 61, 391–9.
17. Eisenberg, E., Carr, D. B. and Chalmers, T. C. (1995) Neurolytic celiac plexus block for treatment of cancer pain: a meta-analysis. *Anesthesia and Analgesia*, 80 (2), 290–5.

4

Pain Clinic procedures

J. F. Hazelgrove and C. Price

Background

Pain Clinics were originally founded as nerve block clinics to treat acute and chronic pain. After the 1939–1945 war the introduction of lignocaine and phenol had a major impact on the techniques used to treat intractable pain.[1] Injection therapy formed the mainstay in the treatment of chronic pain at that time. However, since the 1960s it has been recognized that it should not be used in isolation but as part of an integrated pain management service. In addition, as de-afferentation pain secondary to many of the neurolytic procedures became more widespread, the use of neural blockade became less popular. Therefore, although injection therapy is still widely used, its importance has diminished.

There is much uncertainty about the role of injection therapy, and even more about how it works. The effect of a pain relieving injection can last well beyond the drug's known pharmacological duration. The seventeenth century theories of Descartes suggested that is there is a simple, direct, hard-wired nervous system that is easy to trace and treat. The nervous system is not that simple! The gate control theory postulated that spinal gates in the spinal cord allowed transmission of impulses from pain, temperature and touch fibres into the central nervous system, with descending modulation from the higher central nervous system.[2] Injection therapy is perhaps based upon the premise that blockade of impulses into the central nervous system allows the gates to be shut that were previously open and functioning abnormally. However, this fails to take into account the influence of higher centres and the plasticity of the central nervous system. Thus, nerve blocks tend to be short-lived in effect. It may be possible that short-term pain relief may lead to long-term behavioural change.

Classification of procedures

Injections are performed in the Pain Clinic for three main reasons:

1 Diagnosis
2 Prognosis
3 Therapy

Diagnostic blocks (see Tables 4.1 and 4.2)

Diagnostic blocks are performed in order to try to identify the source of the pain by injecting local anaesthetic. It is important that the needle should be placed precisely. Therefore, knowledge of the anatomy involved is essential, together with fluoroscopy, and contrast or use of a nerve stimulator should be considered. The smallest amount of local anaesthetic necessary should be used. Memory of the effect of a procedure is often very poor in chronic pain sufferers. Patients are therefore asked to record their pain in a diary for the next few days or until the effects wear off.

Problems with diagnostic blocks

Chronic pain is a complex mixture of pain, other abnormal nervous system functioning and outside influences such as emotional, legal, financial and social issues. Therefore, it is unsurprising that diagnostic blocks often fail to give useful information.

Three false assumptions are often made:[3]

- Pathology is located in a precise place.
- Injection of local anaesthetic will block all sensory function.
- Relief of pain after blockade is due to blockade of the neural pathway.

Psychosocial factors that limit diagnostic nerve block include:

- Poor/difficult communication.
- Stress and anxiety altering pain behaviour (e.g. ongoing legal action).
- Differing end-goals between doctor and patient.

The placebo effect may also be important. The probability of response to a placebo injection is proportional to the intensity of the pain. No personality characteristics will predict a placebo response, and most people will respond to a placebo eventually.[4]

To ensure that diagnostic blocks are used with success, there are several points to consider:

- The patient has a diagnosis known to respond to sensory blockade.
- Patient's problems are fully evaluated.
- The operator knows how to block the nerve accurately and treat any complications.
- The nature of the diagnostic block is thoroughly explained to the patient. The patient must understand how to interpret the result. A negative response to a diagnostic block does not mean that the pain is imaginary.
- It is preferable to repeat the block.

Prognostic blocks

The idea of a prognostic injection is to give the doctor and patient some idea of what to expect from a therapeutic block. Unfortunately they are

Table 4.1 Pain Clinic procedures: somatic nerve blocks

Procedure	Common indications	Agents commonly used	Typical volumes used	Specific complications
Epidurals —Lumbar —Thoracic —Cervical —Caudal	Nerve root pain Crush fracture of vertebra	Local anaesthetics Steroids Opioids Adjuvants (ketamine, clonidine)	10–20 ml 10–20 ml 3–5 ml 20 ml	Headache Total spinal Toxic reaction (see text) Hypotension Urinary retention
Facet joint blocks	Mechanical low back pain	Local anaesthetics Steroids Cryotherapy Radiofrequency	0.5–2 ml/h	Motor nerve blockade or damage
Intrathecal injection Intrathecal infusion	Malignant pain	Local anaesthetics Steroids Clonidine Opioids	0.5–2 mls/h	Hypotension Urinary retention Itching Nausea Arachnoiditis Infection

Table 4.2 Pain Clinic procedures: autonomic blocks

Procedure	Indication	Drugs	Volume	Complications
Stellate ganglion	Sympathetically maintained pain (SMP) Upper limb Face Raynaud's Hyperhidrosis	Local anaesthetic	5–10 ml	Vertebra; artery injection Intrathecal injection Hoarse voice Eyelid drop
Lumbar sympathectomy	Vascular insufficiency Lower leg SMP Raynaud's	Local anaesthetic Phenol	5–10 ml	Genitofemoral neuralgia Renal damage
Intrapleural block	Pancreatitic pain Chest wall pain Rib fractures Upper limb SMP	Local anaesthetic	20 ml	Pneumothorax Local anaesthetic Toxicity Horner's Syndrome
Coeliac plexus block	Pancreatitic pain Malignant visceral pain	Local anaesthetic Alcohol	40–50 ml	Local Pain Diarrhoea Hypotension
Intravenous regional blockade	SMP of upper or lower limbs	Local anaesthetic Guanethidine	0.5 mg/kg 0.25 mg/kg	Cuff failure – toxicity Hypotension Stuffy nose Headache

frequently not an accurate reflection of this! Often a prognostic block will apparently succeed only for the surgical treatment to fail. A negative prognostic block does, however, predict failure of a therapeutic block.[5] For this reason it is essential to do a prognostic block before a more permanent procedure is done. They are also useful in convincing the patient of the futility of a more permanent procedure.

To improve the likely success of a prognostic block the same principles should be followed as for diagnostic blockade.

Therapeutic blocks

Therapeutic blocks can be classified into non-neurolytic and neurolytic. The aim is to treat the cause of the pain either completely or as an adjunct to other pain-relieving measures.

Non-neurolytic blockade

- **Local anaesthetics**. Local anaesthetics blocks often have a therapeutic effect lasting long after the pharmacological effect. However, continuous infusions via a catheter are longer acting and more useful.
- **Steroids**. Corticosteroids increase the duration of action of local anaesthetic. They block C-fibres directly and reversibly in intact nerves and neuromas.[6]
- **Opioids**. These are most frequently used with local anaesthetic infusions as they have a synergistic effect.
- **Other**. Other adjuvants used in injections, particularly neuroaxial injections, are ketamine, clonidine and baclofen. These all have slightly different effects and combinations at reduced doses may be useful in limiting side-effects from any one drug.

Neurolytic procedures

- **Alcohol**. This acts by lipid extraction and protein precipitation.[7] It is most commonly used in coeliac plexus blockade and intrathecally. It is hypobaric and therefore patients must be placed with the affected side uppermost if performing an intrathecal injection. It is supplied as 50% or 100% alcohol.
- **Phenol**. This coagulates proteins.[8] It is hyperbaric and therefore patients must be placed with the affected side downwards if performing intrathecal injection. It is supplied as 6% in water or 9% in 60% glycol.
- **Heat and cold (radiofrequency)**. Radiofrequency wave generation acts as a heat sink that coagulates the nerves. Radiofrequency lesions are more precise than solutions of neurolytic agents and rely on localization of the correct nerve fibres by 100 Hz sensory stimulation. After verification that low frequency stimulation does not produce motor root signs the radiofrequency lesion is made. Special needles are used – usually Sluyter Mehta needles. Its long-term outcome is yet to be

established. Cordotomy can be performed using a percutaneous technique with radiofrequency lesioning. It is highly effective in ablating pain pathways for 12–24 months. After this time re-afferentation may occur, which is excruciating for both doctor and patient. It tends to be used in those with a limited life expectancy.

- **Heat and cold (cryotherapy)**. Cryotherapy causes nerve injury by freezing the nerves. It is unclear how exactly it works although it is known that intracellular and extracellular ice crystals are formed.[9] The nerve fibre undergoes Wallerian degeneration. The size of the lesion is dependent on temperature. Regeneration occurs in about 35 days.[10] Neuromas do not occur. It is unclear whether de-afferentation pain occurs after these.

The attendant's role during injection procedures

The role of the attendant (often a nurse) during injection procedures cannot be overstated. Patients have been subjected to a panoply of procedures to minimal effect previously and are naturally apprehensive about what is about to occur. They may also be intimidated by the equipment involved, e.g. X-rays, monitors, needles, etc. The nurse plays an important part in allaying anxiety, explaining what is about to occur and helping the patient to tolerate the procedure. Simultaneously the nurse should be familiar enough with the procedure to help with positioning the patient and to assist the physician.

General advice for all patients undergoing procedures

Most Pain Clinic procedures are done on a day case basis. Therefore guidelines for day surgery units also apply to these patients.[11] However,

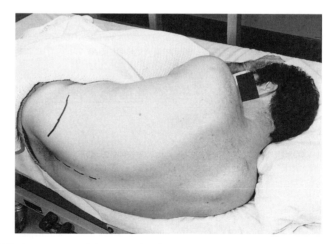

Figure 4.1 Patient positioned for an epidural injection

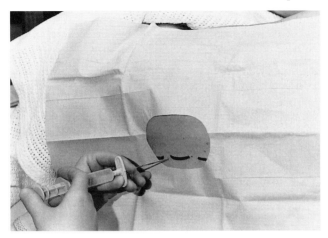

Figure 4.2 An epidural injection being performed

chronic pain patients often have multiple coexisting problems, are elderly or have cancer. Many procedures cause little if any, morbidity. Therefore overnight admission should not be mandatory for these patients.

Before procedures

- Duration of fasting. No food for 6 hours and no drinks for 2 hours before any block associated with serious morbidity, or where sedation may be given.
- Normal medication to be taken. Anticoagulant therapy should be adjusted beforehand.
- A brief medical history, a list of current medications and allergies should be taken.

After the procedure

- All patients should be accompanied home and for the next 24 hours.
- A contact number should be given.
- A note of pain relief if any should be made for the next appointment.
- All current painkillers should be continued unless the patient is specifically told to do otherwise.

Diabetes

If undergoing a corticosteroid injection then abnormally high sugars are more likely. If greater than 5 mmol above usual blood sugar then the patient should contact their GP.

General guidelines

Resuscitation

Many Pain Clinic procedures involve injection of drugs around vessels or into the central nervous system. Misplacement into these structures or allergy may lead to cardiorespiratory collapse. Sedation and X-ray contrast material may cause similar problems. It is therefore essential to ensure that full resuscitation facilities are immediately available and an intravenous cannula should also be placed in most patients.

Radiological protection

All staff involved in procedures requiring an image intensifier should be aware of the problems posed by the use of X-rays and contrast material.[12] The person responsible for the procedure should be appropriately qualified and ensure that all staff have adequate protection. Dosimeters should always be used. Patients should be asked about allergy to iodine-containing substances (iohexol is generally used as contrast material) and in women of child-bearing age the date of the last menstrual period should be sought.

General contraindications to nerve blockade

Injection techniques should not be done if there is a coagulopathy or local sepsis at the point of injection.

General complications of nerve blockade

- Local anaesthetic toxicity (see Figure 4.3).
- Sepsis at the site.
- Intrathecal injection.

Specific procedures in the Pain Clinic

Epidural injection

Common indications

- Radicular pain.
- Pain due to crush fracture/vertebral collapse.
- Spinal stenosis.
- Long term by infusion for cancer pain of lower trunk/limbs.

Positioning

- Lateral or sitting.

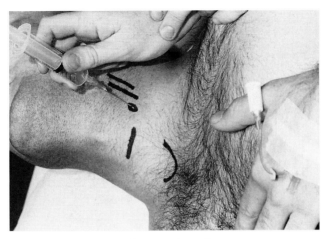

Figure 4.3 A stellate ganglion injection being performed

X-rays required?

- Not usually, unless difficulty is anticipated or a high dose of steroid is injected.

Complications

- Accidental intravenous injection (see algorithm in Figure 4.4).
- Accidental intrathecal injection (see algorithm in Figure 4.5).
- Dural puncture.
- Motor blockade.
- Urinary retention.

Warn the patient

- There may be weakness and/or tingling in their arms or legs depending on where the epidural was placed. This may last 4–6 hours.
- The back of the hand may be sore (site of cannula).
- Pain may increase over the next few days and they should take usual painkillers.
- If they experience a headache that is better when lying flat they should contact the GP or Pain Clinic.

Facet joint injection

These may be diagnostic or therapeutic and involve injections either into the xygo-apophyseal joints of adjacent vertebrae or blockade of the

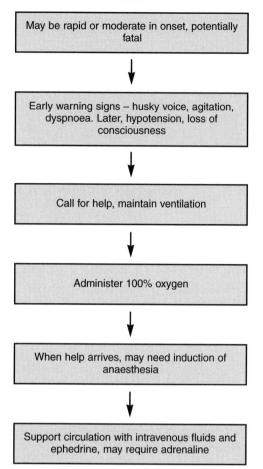

Figure 4.4 Management of total spinal blockade

medial branch of the dorsal ramus that supply these joints. In the former case local anaesthetic with steroid is injected or cryotherapy is performed, in the latter usually diagnostic blocks are followed by radiofrequency lesioning if a positive response is obtained. They may be done anywhere along the spine.

Common indications

Lumbar:

- Low back pain.

Cervical:

- Whiplash syndrome.
- Neck pain or cervicogenic headache due to arthritis in those joints.

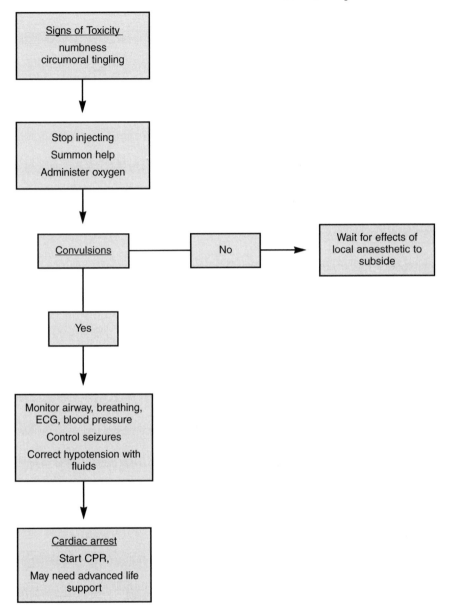

Figure 4.5 Treatment of local anaesthetic toxicity

Positioning

• Prone with pillow underneath to allow flexion of spine.

X-rays required?

• Yes.

Complications

Lumbar:

- Accidental motor root injection (rare).

Cervical:

- Accidental motor root injection (rare).
- Vertebral artery injection.
- Ataxia (particularly higher joints).

Warn the patient

- To expect some weakness in a leg, which will wear off within 24 hours.
- To avoid lifting or strenous tasks but try gentle mobility to increase flexibility.

If cryoanalgesia to the joint has been performed the patient should be warned to expect:

- A temporary increase in pain or tingling.
- If there is any inflammation around the site then the patient should see their GP.

If radiofrequency lesions of the joints have been performed then the patient should be warned:

- Pain may worsen before it gets better or there may be tingling or paraesthesia in the buttock, legs or back for lumbar facets and shoulder or neck for cervical facets.

Stellate ganglion block

The stellate ganglion is in the neck and is near to the vertebral artery, trachea, lung and epidural space. This should be remembered when this block is done!

Common indications

- Complex Regional Pain Syndrome type I of the upper limb, face.
- Raynaud's syndrome.
- Sympathetically mediated pain of the upper limb.

Positioning

- Supine.

X-rays required?

- No.

Complications

- Accidental intravascular injection leading to convulsions (see algorithm in Figure 4.4).
- Intrathecal injection (see algorithm in Figure 4.5).
- Pneumothorax.
- Horner's syndrome, an inevitable complication.
- Hoarse voice.

Warn the patient

- Throat may be bruised and may have a hoarse voice.
- Eyelid may droop.
- Cheek may be hotter on that side.
- Arm may be weak.
- May have a stuffy nose.
- May get short of breath. If this has been performed as an outpatient procedure the patient should then seek medical advice.

Coeliac plexus blockade

This is an injection around the coeliac plexus, which is situated around the aorta in the upper abdomen. The block may be with local anaesthetic as a diagnostic block or as a neurolytic block when 50 ml of 50% alcohol is used. Usually the patient is prone, although if difficulty is anticipated the procedure may be done with CT guidance.

Common indications

- Pancreatitis, chronic.
- Visceral pain of any origin.

Positioning

- Prone.
- Arms lifted up onto the pillow.

X-rays required?

- Yes, with contrast medium. May be done with a CT-guided approach although this is logistically quite difficult to do.

Complications

- Local pain relief.
- Diarrhoea.
- Hypotension.
- Haematoma.
- Impotence.

Lumbar sympathectomy

Lumbar sympathectomy may be diagnostic or therapeutic. If therapeutic then either phenol or alcohol is used.

Common indications

- Palliation of pain due to vascular insufficiency.
- Post-herpetic neuralgia.
- Sympathetically maintained pain of the lower extremities.

Positioning

- The patient should be placed in the lateral position with the side to be blocked uppermost. A pillow should be placed underneath the flank.

X-rays required?

- Yes, with contrast medium.

Complications

- Damage to kidney.
- Accidental epidural injection.
- Trauma to nerve roots.
- Discitis.
- Pneumothorax.
- Genitofemoral neuralgia.
- Postural hypotension.

Warn the patient

- Warm leg.
- Sore back.
- May feel light headed if sat up.
- May experience groin pain, which is usually temporary.

Intercostal nerve block

This block may be diagnostic, therapeutic or prognostic and single or multiple blocks may be performed. At least three should be done as the area of pain is served by the nerves above and below as well.

Common indications

- Evaluation of chest wall pain.
- With local anaesthetic as a prognostic indicator of more permanent block.

- Palliation of chest wall pain.
- Post-herpetic neuralgia in that area.

Note that even if there is a coagulopathy this block can be so effective in palliative care it is worth doing.

Positioning

- Prone, sitting or lateral.

X-rays required?

- If neurolytic procedure is to be done, with contrast medium.

Complications

- Pneumothorax.
- Intravascular injection.

Warn the patient

- If they become short of breath to contact an emergency department and give details of the procedure.

Guanethidine blockade

This involves a Bier's block, injection of guanethidine and a tourniquet applied for 20 minutes. Two cannulae need to be inserted, one in the affected limb and one elsewhere. It is often a good idea to place the affected limb in warm water beforehand.

Common indications

- Complex Regional Pain Syndrome type I of a limb.
- Other sympathetically maintained pain of the limb.

Contraindications

- Sickle cell disease.
- Uncontrolled hypertension or angina.

Positioning

- Reclining.

X-rays required?

- No.

Complications

- Accidental tourniquet deflation.
- Headache.
- Stuffy nose.
- Hypertension.
- Postural hypotension.
- Arrhythmias (rare).

Spinal cord stimulation

Spinal cord stimulation involves electrical stimulation of the dorsal columns which relay pain messages in the spinal cord. Electrodes are placed in the epidural space near to the dorsal column under X-ray control. Sedation is inevitably required. Electrical impulses modulate the pain messages in the dorsal columns. They may also dilate blood vessels. As they are implantable devices a commitment to long-term care is essential. They may become infected, wires break or the device fail. They should therefore only be done by those who are experienced in their use. Also, continued support, ongoing physiotherapy and careful explanations as to how to use the stimulator are necessary.

Common indications

- Angina.
- Peripheral vascular disease.
- Complex Regional Pain Syndromes.
- Failed Back Syndrome with radicular pain.

X-rays required?

- Yes.

Positioning

- Prone.

Complications

- Slippage.
- Fracture of wires.
- Infection.

Summary
- A vast number of procedures may be carried out in the Pain Clinic.
- Many of these procedures are useful in the management of cancer pains refractory to other treatments.
- Evidence is lacking for long-term benefit of many of the procedures in cases of chronic pain.
- Procedures should be carried out as part of a multidisciplinary strategy to manage the pain in the long term.
- Intravenous access and full resuscitation facilities should be readily available, with staff trained to recognize and treat the life-threatening events that may occur.
- Local guidelines should be in operation to ensure the safe discharge of these patients on the same day of their treatment.

References

1. Bonica, J. J. (1990) *The Management of Pain*, 2nd edn. Media: Lea & Febiger.
2. Melzack, R. and Wall, P. D. (1965) Pain mechanisms: a new theory. *Science*, 150, 971–9.
3. Cousins, M. J. (1998) *Pain Neural Blockade in Clinical Anesthesia and Management of Pain.* Philadelphia: Lippincott–Raven.
4. McQuay, H. and Moore, A. (1998) *An Evidence Based Source of Pain Relief.* Oxford: Oxford University Press.
5. North, R. B., Kidd, D. H., Zahurak, M. and Piantadosi, S. (1996) Specificity of diagnostic nerve blocks: a prospective, randomized study of sciatica due to lumbosacral disease. *Pain*, 65, 77–85.
6. Devor, M., Govrin-Lippmann, R. and Raber, P. (1985) Corticosteroids suppress ectopic discharge originating in experimental neuromas. *Pain*, 22, 127–37.
7. Rumsby, M. G. and Finean, J. B. (1966) The action of organic solvents on the myelin nerve sheath of peripheral nerve tissue: II Short-chain aliphatic alcohols. *Journal of Neurochemistry*, 13, 1509–11.
8. Wood, K. M. (1978) The use of phenol as a neurolytic agent: a review. *Pain*, 5, 205–29.
9. Evans, P. J. D., Lloyd, J. W. and Green, C. J. (1981) Cryoanalgesia: the response to alteration in freeze cycle and temperature. *British Journal of Anaesthesia*, 53, 1121–7.
10. Kalichman, M. W. and Myers, R. R. (1987) Behavioral and electrophysiological recovery following cryogenic nerve injury. *Experimental Neurology*, 96, 692–702.
11. Royal College of Surgeons (1993) *Guidelines for Day-Case Surgery.* London: RCS.
12. Department of Health (1988) *The Ionising Radiation (Protection of Persons Undergoing Medical Examination or Treatment) Regulations.* London: HMSO.

5

Malignant pain: cancer pain

P. Pitcher and C. Duncombe

Introduction

This chapter will define the nature and extent of chronic malignant pain so that the reader may show an appreciation of all its components. It is important to understand in the broadest terms the impact on the patient, family and health care professional of chronic malignant pain and understand the significance of, and skills required for, pain assessment.

Chronic malignant pain is not a commonly used term and encompasses two important components. The first of these is the word 'chronic'. This has been defined as pain lasting 3 months or more.[1] Malignant has been described both sociologically and medically:

- disposed to do harm, actuated by great hatred and tending to cause death or to go from bad to worse.[2]
- mass of cells that is capable of metastasizing and can threaten the host's survival;[3] in other words, cancer.

It might, therefore, be assumed that chronic malignant pain could be described as pain caused by or related to cancer, with a duration of 3 months or more. However, the picture is more complex than this. Some people with cancer will not survive as long as 3 months from diagnosis. That is not to say that symptoms have only been present for 3 months; indeed, even at presentation, patients may have had symptoms for some time. For the patients themselves the time duration may be meaningless. The patient's personal experience and the way that others respond to that experience may be more significant to the way that an individual describes their pain. Indeed, when facing a life-threatening disease it may be questionable whether categorizing pain into acute and chronic is beneficial to the patient. A new acute pain on top of existing cancer pain requires the same approach and palliative management. In addition, it should be noted that the concept of chronic pain is broader than just a temporal component and encompasses peripheral responses of the organism and central nervous modifications.

However, detailed discussion of this is outside the scope of this chapter. For clarity in this chapter, chronic malignant pain will be referred to broadly as cancer pain. For many patients a diagnosis of cancer means certain pain. This is not necessarily the case; up to one-third of patients with cancer will never experience pain.[4]

It is vital to consider the widest possible view of a patient's cancer pain. McCaffrey's definition of pain as 'pain is what the patient says it is and exists whenever he or she says it does'[5] will be very familiar to nurses. This same concept has been described in palliative medicine: 'Pain is a somatopsychic experience best defined as "what the subject says hurts".'[4] Both of these quotes illustrate the importance of considering the personal, subjective and unique experience of every individual's pain. Fordham and Dunn add that 'pain is known by others only when information about it is communicated by the one experiencing it. Knowing by others is once removed.'[6] This pain experience has many facets and includes physical, spiritual, psychological, cultural and social aspects. It is also important to remember that patients may have more than one pain: Only one-fifth of patients have just one pain. Some four-fifths have two or more pains and one-third have four pains or more.[4] Cancer pain may be associated with both the disease process or the treatment, and often there is pre-existing pain not related to the cancer at all. Previous experience of pain, be it personal or that of other people, how people have reacted to that pain, and the potential meaning of the pain to the person, can influence the current pain experience. Importantly, these issues are just as relevant to the health care professional interpreting that pain. Indeed, the nurse cannot divorce him- or herself from the process of pain management. Who we are as human beings, the experiences that make us what and who we are, as well as the values that we hold are highly significant. These important factors influence the way in which we react to patients' pain, report that pain and, subsequently, the way in which we manage it. All these points begin to illustrate both the subjective nature and complexity of the cancer pain experience. This chapter will explore these issues in more detail.

The meaning of pain

For the nurse caring for the patient in pain, an understanding of what that pain means to each individual patient is vital. Where this understanding is absent, there may be a disparity in the patient and nurse's approach to pain management. We need to reflect on the fact that pain may mean different things to different patients and indeed in the same patients at different times. Consider the difference between the pain of childbirth and, say, the pain of widespread pelvic tumour invading a nerve pathway. For the woman experiencing labour there is the knowledge that it will come to an end, that it is not harmful and that it will normally produce a happy outcome. The malignant pelvic pain may not be as severe, but may be unremitting and a constant reminder of impending death and many associated losses. When assessing cancer patients' pain it may be very useful to simply ask, 'What does this pain mean to you?' Similarly, it may be helpful to ask the patient of their previous experience of cancer. This previous experience may be on a personal level, but may be associated with seeing others with cancer in pain. Older patients may have very negative memories of parents dying of cancer in severe pain. This is often compounded by the fact that the experience of bereavement may influence our perception, so that we remember the pain as being more severe than it was in reality. Attention to these factors is important to unpack these broader perceptions and expectations in order to fully understand each patient's pain experience. Many patients will perceive their pain as more severe if it lacks positive meaning and has no expected end except death. Intractable pain is often found in patients in whom mental and social factors are ignored. Nurses need to remember that a patient's pain tolerance is affected not only by meaning but also by mood and morale. Attention to these factors gives the patient, family and health care professional significant assistance in managing cancer pain.

Readers may find it helpful to stop and consider their own pain experiences. Ask yourself: 'What were my earliest memories of pain?', 'How was that pain reacted to?', 'How do I feel now when I have pain?', 'What do I feel about other people's pain?', 'Do I have a high pain tolerance?' and so on. Reflect on your answers and how they might influence the values that you have developed professionally. Most of us would like to feel that we have a high pain tolerance; many of us may consider others to have a lower pain tolerance. What do we mean by this? How have we measured this? Do we consider it to be worthy to be able to tolerate high levels of pain? It is important to remember that pain is such a subjective experience, and only the patient is qualified to truly describe that pain. If, for example, ten nurses all scored their back pain out of ten and all scored the same, we could never know whether their pains were all the same. For the nurse developing skills in pain assessment and management this is a vital concept to understand.

Apart from our personal experience of pain there is the effect of our professional experience. In a study of nurses working in a burns unit patients were asked to score their pain out of ten. Nurses were then independently asked to score the same patient's pain, again out of ten. The two sets of results were compared. Nurses who had worked in this burns unit the longest tended to score the patients' pain lower than the patients themselves. Newer and less experienced nurses tended to either score the same as the patients or even higher than the patients.[7] What could be the explanation for this? Is it that when we are constantly exposed to unacceptable levels of pain we tend to distance ourselves and underestimate the severity of patients' pain in order to make our jobs tolerable? Is it easier to accept that a person's pain is not as bad as they may say it is than to have to accept that we are surrounded by distressed patients whom we may feel unable to help?

Skills of assessment

To assess a patient's pain, we must take the whole suffering process into account or the non-physical elements of pain will go unrecognized and unaddressed. This concept of recognizing the entire suffering process is often called total pain.[8]

Skilled assessment is the cornerstone of effective pain management. The aim of assessment is to identify the individual nature and extent of the pain experience for each patient. Accurate assessment results in many advantages for both the patient and health care professional (Table 5.1):

Table 5.1 Advantages of accurate pain assessment

Patient	Health care professional
Helps achieve quickest possible symptom control	Helps establish a good working relationship with patient
Patient feels listened to and heard	Ensures effective time management
Minimizes undesirable side-effects	Avoids wasting resources
Addresses concept of total pain	Aids professional development and experience
	Accurate targeting of pain control

It also needs to be remembered that for many patients, pain has been the presenting symptom and may be accompanied by other frightening symptoms, for example, breathlessness. Indeed 30% of cancer patients are already in pain when their disease is diagnosed.[9] The process of pain assessment relies on a range of skills and knowledge. Many of these skills nurses will already possess: these include listening and observation, and knowledge of types of pain and their relation to the disease process. These skills need to be developed, as does a sound knowledge of drugs used in pain management. For example, if a patient tells the nurse that his immediate release morphine solution is providing relief for 4 hours, the nurse needs to be aware that this is normal for this preparation, and not draw the conclusion that the analgesia is ineffective and needs changing.

A range of questions and observations needs to be considered (see Table 5.2). The patient's previous response to analgesia therapies is particularly important. For example, a patient may say that they have tried oramorph (oral, immediate release, morphine sulphate solution) and report that it did not work. On closer questioning the nurse may discover that the patient has only tried one or two doses, possibly with too wide a dose interval or too low a dose. Only through identifying these sorts of issues can a proper therapeutic trial of appropriate analgesia be tried rather than dismissing the analgesia as ineffective.

The use of good listening skills is of great value to the nurse making a pain assessment. The patient who is asked 'Have you got any pain today?' or, even worse, 'You haven't got any pain have you?' may give a very different reply if asked 'How are you feeling today, how is your pain?' By the simple strategy of asking an open question, rather than a closed question, the nurse may elicit much more information. Even the patient who denies pain may have another agenda. Are they afraid of being given a strong painkiller? After all, for many patients, being given morphine may be seen as the beginning of the end. Conversely, patients may not be keen to admit that their pain is better. This may be because

Table 5.2 Pain assessment: questions and observations

- Where is the pain? Describe its nature, severity, location, duration, precipitating factors and any temporal pattern.
- Is there more than one pain?
- Are there associated signs and symptoms? E.g. swelling, nausea, numbness and tingling.
- Are there metastases? Potential cause: where is the primary malignancy? What common patterns might it follow?
- How has the pain responded to previous analgesic therapies? E.g. if there has been a response to analgesia, which type, how long does it last and how much of the pain does it resolve?
- What non-pharmacological measures (if any) relieve the pain?
- Are there non-malignant pain problems? E.g. constipation, arthritis
- Does the pain interfere with the patient's activities of daily living?

---

they fear being abandoned once their pain is under control. Nurses use skills of visual observation all the time. In pain assessment this is an important part of the process:

- Does the patient grimace when moved?
- Are certain activities avoided?
- How well does the patient mobilize?
- Is what the patient says congruent with facial expression?
- Is the patient pale and sweaty?

Observing the patient's ability to be distracted or to engage in normal activities also helps us to assess their level of pain.

Use of pain charts in assessment

Pain charts can be a useful adjunct in any pain assessment for some patients. However, it is important to remember that they cannot replace the above skills but may be a tool to add to them. The foundation of effective pain management remains the relationship between the nurse and the patient – in our experience this is particularly true in cancer pain, with all the underlying issues which this diagnosis raises which can render the pain experience more complex.

Pain charts used in the assessment of cancer pain usually consist of several elements to reflect this complexity. A body chart is often included, which may be particularly useful when the patient themselves fills in the area(s) affected by pain. The chronic nature of cancer pain means that this kind of record can be kept as a pain history to aid assessment over a longer period of time. In addition, some kind of quantification of the pain is often included, whether in the form of a visual analogue or a verbal rating scale. Qualities of the pain in the form of descriptors (e.g. burning, shooting, constant) can also be useful to help establish the nature and cause of the pain. Two other elements documented in assessment charts for cancer pain may be precipitating and relieving factors and, finally, mood.[10] An important element in the use of pain charts is the value of ongoing assessment, which can be a delicate balance in cancer pain management. Whilst a one-off assessment is of little value, so also may be very frequent assessments of the detailed nature described above. The latter can serve to focus attention on a chronic problem that may be slow to resolve or may prove intractable which can, in turn, compound the pain experience.[10] The frequency of ongoing assessment using pain charts is therefore an individual matter requiring negotiation between the patient and the nurse.

There are some problems with using detailed pain charts in cancer pain assessment that may account for their variable use. For some patients, attempting to quantify their pain is a very difficult task; what did the score of 5 yesterday actually feel like? We can ask ourselves the same kind of question: 'How does my headache feel today compared to the last one I had?' Pain charts may also prove less useful when patients do not wish to have responsibility for their own pain management, preferring to leave it to the health care professionals. Other problems can include staff lack of confidence in being able to improve the patient's pain and, therefore, a reticence about using detailed formal assessment that highlights the problem; lack of realistic goals set in conjunction with the patient in complex pain situations may compound this lack of confidence.

Pain charts can, therefore, be a useful aid to cancer pain assessment, although they do have drawbacks. Importantly, the elements helpful to the individual patient can be taken individually, and used either formally or informally. For example, the patient may find filling in a body chart helpful or may prefer simply indicating to the nurse where the pain is. The same is true for rating scales, exacerbating and relieving factors, and mood. If the assessment is informal it becomes the nurse's responsibility to ensure accurate documentation of the information to maintain continuity of care.

Types of cancer pain

As identified earlier, patients with cancer may experience many types of pain. It is therefore important to distinguish these to enable accurate treatment to be instigated. In a survey of 211 patients with pain, carried out at Michael Sobell House in Oxford, UK, the 10 most frequent causes of pain could be identified (Table 5.3). Some of the categories may be surprising.

It can be seen from Table 5.3 that not all pain suffered by cancer patients is a direct result of the cancer itself. In addition, it needs to be remembered that some malignant diseases result in more pain than others and a knowledge of the common cancers and the associated pain incidence is important.

In order to understand the wide spectrum of cancer pain and aid assessment it may be useful to consider four main categories:

- pain associated with tumour involvement.
- pain indirectly due to cancer.
- pain due to cancer therapy.
- pain independent of cancer.

Table 5.3 Ten most common causes of pain in cancer patient

Nature of pain	Cause
Bone	Cancer
Nerve compression	Cancer
Soft tissue	Cancer
Visceral	Cancer
Myofascial	Debility
Constipation	Debility
Muscle spasm	Cancer/Debility
Low back pain	Concurrent disorders
Chronic postoperative	Treatment
Capsulitis of shoulder	Debility

Source: Data from Twycross, R. G. and Lack, S. A. (1990).[4]

Pain associated with tumour involvement

This category is the most common type of pain in cancer patients, and occurs when a tumour infiltrates, stretches or presses on an organ or nerve. Examples include tumour infiltration of bone (for example, metastases from lung, prostate or breast), pancoast tumour (where there is direct invasion of the brachial plexus causing severe pain) and fungating breast lesions (where there is erosion and destruction of soft tissue).

Pain indirectly due to cancer

This type of pain is due to the debility associated with advancing cancer

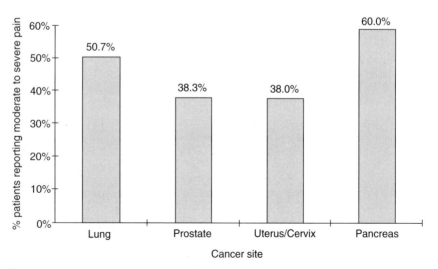

Figure 5.1 Prevalence of cancer pain. (After Greenwald, H. P., Bonica, J. J. and Bergner, M. (1987)[11]

and includes tissue damage such as pressure sores and joint and muscle pain from immobility and muscle wasting. Acute herpetic and post-herpetic neuralgia can occur in this patient population because cancer patients have five times the incidence of infection with varicella-zoster.[12]

Pain due to cancer therapy

This category has been estimated to account for 19% of pain in an inpatient population and 25% in an outpatient population.[12] This covers the wide range of cancer treatment, including surgery, chemotherapy and radiotherapy. Examples include post-thoracotomy pain, post-mastectomy pain syndrome and phantom limb (or other organ amputation) pain, but this is covered elsewhere in this book, and peripheral neuropathy and musculoskeletal pain, in particular jaw, after vincristine therapy and some other chemotherapy agents. Oral mucositis is a common pain syndrome in patients receiving intensive chemotherapy. Post-radiation pain is less common, but may be seen when there is damage to a peripheral nerve or the spinal cord and often occurs late in the course of the illness. Radiation fibrosis of the brachial plexus and radiation myelopathy are specific examples. Treatment of certain cancer pains may result in other pain; for example, the use of strong opioids may result in constipation and associated pain and discomfort.

Pain independent of cancer

This needs to be mentioned because patients with cancer are still subject to the range of aches and pains that affect the general population, but none the less still need addressing. Indeed, the majority of patients with cancer are elderly and therefore more likely to have pre-existing degenerative conditions. The commonest examples are osteoarthritis, angina and migraine. Many of these pains may be worsened because of stress, anxiety and immobility.

The impact of cancer pain on the patient, family and health care professional

The impact of the pain associated with cancer on the patient and all those around the patient cannot be overestimated. A diagnosis of cancer inevitably results in many emotional and psychological difficulties; many patients describe a 'rollercoaster' of emotional responses. Pain may be intimately involved in the patient's experience in two ways. First, there is the impact of the pain itself on the patient and family, including fear, anxiety, loss of role, loss of independence, depression and immobility. Secondly, there is the way in which all the emotional responses to cancer and other stresses may impact on the pain itself, often worsening the pain and complicating the treatment. From these two points it can be seen that pain can add to the patient's emotional burden, but that also the emotional state of the patient can equally contribute to the pain picture. Commonly, both occur, producing a difficult cyclical effect. Clearly the nurse caring for the patient in pain cannot separate the emotional and psychological issues. Cicely Saunders, widely held to be the founder of the modern hospice movement, developed the concept of 'total pain', which encompasses physical, social, psychological and spiritual factors when managing cancer patients in pain.[13] Patients who fail to respond to conventional analgesia regimes need careful reassessment with particular attention to *all factors*, in particular the psychosocial component. It is important not to fall into the familiar trap of describing patients' pain as 'psychosomatic' or 'all in the mind' and the subsequent judgements and dismissals that we have all seen. It is rare that pain is either all physical or all psychological, and even where the pain is felt to be of a mainly psychological origin it must carry equal weight and value as any obviously physically based pain. Patients whose pain has a strong psychosocial element still need our skills and expertise in management.

> *Pauline was a 49-year-old woman with cancer of the ovary. She had a senior position in a major recruitment company and presented as a typically high-powered, successful businesswoman: smart, efficient and extremely busy, she had no time for cancer in her life. Pauline had undergone surgical excision 6 months previously, had made a fairly uneventful postoperative recovery and had been working until the day prior to admission.*
>
> *Accompanied by her husband, Daniel, she was admitted to a general surgical ward as an emergency in severe pain. Despite several doses of pethidine, her pain worsened. The Hospital Palliative Care Team was asked to see her immediately. When the Clinical Nurse Specialist from the team arrived he found an extremely distressed woman in severe pain. She was literally screaming out and writhing around the bed complaining of severe shooting pain in her left hip. With help from her husband she was able to tell her story. She had had increasing poor health and pain over the past 6 weeks. When asked about her family she described her much loved son who had been a soldier in Northern Ireland, where he had met and married an Irish woman. At the end of his term of service in the army he had been very strongly advised not to settle in Belfast. However, under pressure from his wife's family he had bought a house there, although the army advised him that this could be very dangerous. As Pauline described her fears for her son, her pain visibly worsened and she cried out increasingly. She also went on to describe how she had concealed her cancer from everyone, including her boss and her son.*
>
> *Pauline's pain remained extremely difficult to resolve. However, we encouraged her to talk to her son on the telephone, who then came over to England. Although deeply distressing for them both, they were able to talk to each other about their fears and anxieties as well as the things that mattered to them both. Pauline was helped to tell the people who were close to her what was happening to her and to prepare them for her death. Importantly, enabling Pauline to understand the relationship between her pain and her emotional difficulties helped her to manage her pain more effectively. It was eventually decided that transfer to the hospice would be helpful so that she would have access to expert palliative medical support for symptom control. Furthermore, the hospice was able to support the family more effectively. Although initially very distressed, Pauline was able to be peaceful for the last couple of days of her life and died just over a week after admission.*

There may be underlying issues within the family or within the person that may surface at critical points. These may further affect the pain experience and, again, need sensitive and careful exploration. It is worth remembering that these issues may be so powerful that the pain is never fully controlled. None the less these patients still need the nurse's skill in order to find ways of managing the pain, and the acknowledgement of the issues may in itself be helpful for the patient, family and staff. In particular, the nursing staff who are most closely involved may be enabled to cope with being alongside the patient with uncontrolled pain.

The effects on the family, or others close to the patient but not necessarily related, cannot be overestimated. This further has an impact on the patient's pain. Typically, family members describe feelings of helplessness and inadequacy, and this may manifest itself by them either distancing themselves from the patient or rating the patient's pain more severely than the patient. It can also be difficult for relatives to understand their own emotions at times. They may complain that the patient is in severe pain and that it is not being attended to, but this may be a manifestation of their own despair and sense of helplessness. This can cause some tension between the nursing staff and the relatives. Careful and sensitive exploration of the issues may reveal some of the feelings described above. However, the role of the family in supporting the patient in pain can be very valuable and the nurse has an important role in supporting the family in this task. Enabling the relatives to participate in care where this is appropriate and desired may help to minimize feelings of helplessness. Careful listening, facilitating meaningful communication between the patient and family, and reassuring the relatives of their valuable role, may be helpful to everyone. This is supported by Dar,[14] who highlighted some of the difficulties spouses of cancer patients experience. In particular, patients tend to underestimate the impact of their pain on their spouses.

Other common difficulties that relatives may describe include feelings of anger, anxiety, hopelessness, resentment, role tension, marital conflict, reduced sexual activity and despondency.

Conclusion

This chapter has concentrated on the role of the nurse in cancer pain management. However, it is important to emphasize that effective management is best achieved by collaborative teamwork between the patient, nurse, doctor and other health care professionals. Each has a vital role and perspective to contribute if the management is to be optimal. Teamwork becomes even more important when the pain is refractory to treatment in order that those involved can continue to stay alongside the patient and their family.

Equally, the contribution of specialist teams should be mentioned. Palliative care, acute pain and chronic pain teams can all play a part in supporting patients, families and health care professionals in situations where the staff immediately involved find conventional first-line treatments are not working, or there is doubt about which treatment to pursue.

The nurse working most closely with the patient has a key role in cancer pain management. It is hoped that this chapter has helped to raise awareness of the many potential aspects of the pain experience for this patient population and thereby aid accurate assessment and treatment.

Summary
- Cancer pain is a complex, multifaceted phenomenon.
- Psychological aspects cannot be separated from the pain experience, both for patients and health care professionals.
- Effective management is not about drug therapy alone, but also about attention to all relevant aspects of a person's pain.
- Each nurse needs to start by considering his or her own attitudes to and experience of pain.
- Accurate, comprehensive assessment is the foundation of effective cancer pain management.
- It may not be possible to relieve pain totally, or even partially, in every situation. The nurse still has an important role in supporting the patient and family.

Acknowledgements

We wish to acknowledge, with thanks, our colleague and friend Katherine Penn for her assistance in preparing this chapter.

References

1. Carpenito, L. J. (1983) *Nursing Diagnosis: Application to Clinical Practice*, 4th edn. Philadelphia: J.B. Lippincott.
2. Landau, S. I. (ed.) (1988) *Chambers English Dictionary*. Cambridge: Cambridge University Press.
3. Eriksson, J. H. (1990) *Oncologic Nursing*. London: Springhouse Notes.
4. Twycross, R. G. and Lack, S. A. (1990) *Therapeutics in Terminal Cancer*. Edinburgh: Churchill Livingstone.
5. McCaffrey, M. (1979) *Nursing Management of the Patient with Pain*. Philadelphia: J.B. Lipincott.
6. Fordham, M. and Dunn, V. (1994) *Alongside the Person in Pain: Holistic Care and Nursing Practice*. London: Bailliere Tindall.
7. Choiniere, M., Melzack, R., Girard, N., Rondeau, J. and Paquin, M. J. (1990) Comparisons between patients' and nurses' assessment of pain and medication efficacy in severe burn injuries. *Pain*, 40(2), 143–52.
8. Fallon, M. T. (1995) Transdermal fentanyl in cancer pain. *Journal of Pain and Symptom Management*, 10(2), 87.
9. Livneh, J., Garber, A. and Shaevich, E. (1998) Assessment and documentation of pain in oncology patients. *International Journal of Palliative Nursing*, 4 (4), 169–75.
10. Walker, V.A. and Dicks, B. (1987) Pain assessment charts in the management of chronic cancer pain. *Palliative Medicine*, 1, 111–16.
11. Greenwald, H. P., Bonica, J. J. and Bergner, M. (1987) Prevalence of pain in four cancers. *Cancer*, 60(10), 2563–9.
12. Doyle, D., Hanks, G. W. C. and MacDonald, N. (eds) (1993) *Oxford Textbook of Palliative Medicine*. Oxford: Oxford University Press.
13. Saunders, C. (1967) *The Management of Terminal Illness*. London: Edward Arnold.
14. Dar, R., Beech, C. M., Barden, P. L. and Cleeland, C. S. (1992) Cancer pain in the marital system: a study of patients and their spouses. *Journal of Pain and Symptom Management*, 7(2), 87–93.

6

Non-malignant pain: chronic back pain

S. Thomas

Introduction

This chapter will show that chronic back pain is a major problem for both the individual concerned and for the National Health Service. It is an area where diagnosis can be difficult and individuals may not have a diagnosis for months. McCaffrey[1] defines pain as being 'Whatever the experiencing person says it is and exists whenever the experiencing person says it does.' This definition of pain is often quoted but just as frequently only receives lip service. If there is no obvious diagnosis it can be easy for health care professionals to adopt the view that chronic back pain is psychological or non-existent. However, it is important that the individual is believed.[2] If not, they may become alienated and unwilling to receive advice which could be beneficial. Just by listening and believing the individual when they express pain, this problem can be overcome. During treatment, both conservative and surgical, the individual should feel they are part of the team. This will help reduce anxiety and increase compliance with treatment.

Anatomy and common causes of chronic back pain are briefly addressed. This is not comprehensive, but serves to give an overview into how the spine is constructed and some of the ways in which problems can occur. For more detail in these areas, suggested reading is included.

Chronic pain has been described as pain which lasts for 3 months or longer.[3,4] Methods of pain relief are discussed. There are a variety of treatments that can be utilized, and different methods will affect different people in different ways. We are all unique and have our own experiences and perceptions. If one method of pain relief does not work, try another. It should be remembered that it may not be possible to fully alleviate chronic back pain.

The individual needs education on how to care for their back correctly, as this will aid in the reduction of pain and may assist in the healing of the original cause of the pain. Also, exercises that will help strengthen surrounding muscles should be taught. This will help reduce the pain, as these muscles will assist in supporting the spine and could also aid in the prevention of a new injury.

This chapter will assist the reader in considering a patient-focused view of care, which can be especially effective with those who suffer from chronic back pain. It also gives valuable information that can help the individual to begin to overcome the problems they face.

The cost of chronic back pain

Back pain is a common condition, affecting 80% of adults at some time in their lives.[5] Each year, 4.5% of adults are diagnosed by their general practitioner (GP) as having lower back pain. This means two and a quarter million people consult their GP each year. Three hundred and fifty thousand are referred to hospital outpatient departments, and some 65 000 are admitted to hospital, staying an average of 12 days. It is estimated that 1.5% of the National Health Service (NHS) budget is spent in the treatment of back pain.[6] The same report estimated that back pain accounted for a loss of over 33 million working days, 9.2% of all days lost through certified incapacity. In 90% of cases, recovery will come in the first 4–6 weeks; the remaining 10%, however, take longer. Waddle[7] published more recent figures, showing that over a 20 year period the number of days lost from work increased from around 10 million in 1975 to over 100 million in 1995.

These economic problems are not limited to Britain. In the Netherlands absenteeism due to back pain costs an average of one and a half million dollars per hour[8] and in the USA it is estimated to cost 16 billion dollars a year.[5]

These figures only refer to longer-term conditions and those who have visited their GP, however. They do not show acute problems and those who have not sought a medical opinion. This suggests the total could be much higher. They do clearly indicate a significant impact world wide as well as to the economy of Britain and the NHS.

An area often overlooked is the cost to the individual both economically and socially. Some recent reports continue to leave the reader with the impression that those suffering long-term back pain are eager to collect benefits associated with being sick.[9] Other reports, such as that written by Linton,[8] focus more on the economic difficulties linked with chronic back pain. For those on long-term sick leave, salaries will become affected, leaving the individual on reduced pay or on welfare benefits. Consideration should also be made for social factors. Long-term pain and disability will make it harder to live what is considered a normal life; shopping, for example, may be difficult or impossible. Social contact may decline, leaving more time to reflect upon the pain; this cycle has been described by Braggins.[10] The proposed series of events perpetuating back pain involves the pain leading to reduced activity tolerance, which decreases the level of well-being. This increases the cognitive appraisal of the pain which, in turn, increases the amount of pain felt. The cycle will then repeat. Breaking this cycle is necessary in the treatment of chronic back pain, where a cure is not always achievable. How this may be achieved is discussed later in this chapter.

A little anatomy

The spine, or vertebral column, is a complex structure. It consists of 24 vertebrae and 23 intervertebral discs, held together by muscles and ligaments. There are 7 cervical, 12 thoracic and 5 lumbar vertebrae. Two fused sections, the sacrum and coccyx, also make up part of the structure.

The main functions of the spine include protecting the spinal cord and giving support in transferring loads, from head and arms through to the pelvis. It is highly flexible, allowing a wide range of movement due to the pliable nature of the intervertebral discs. The centre of the disc contains a gelatinous mass known as the nucleus pulposus, and the outer fibrocartilaginous ring is called the annulus fibrosis.

The vertebrae consist of a vertebral body, which is roughly cylindrical in shape and sits between the discs. Bony prominences coming from the posterior aspect of the vertebral body are known as spinous processes. To the anterior aspect of the body are joints known as facets. They enable movement against those facets above and below. The top facet is called the superior articulating facet, as it is above the vertebra. The bottom facet is known as the inferior articulating facet, as it is below the vertebra.

The flexibility provided by the discs and the density of the bone is reduced in ageing. Consequently, the elderly are more susceptible to problems relating to the spine.

For more detailed anatomy and for physiology suggested reading includes Tortora[11] and Brooker.[12]

The main causes of chronic back pain

Pain is a symptom. The individual suffering with chronic back pain will have a problem that is either mechanical or inflammatory. There are many different conditions requiring a variety of treatments so accuracy of diagnosis is essential.

The most common identified problem causing chronic back pain is a prolapsed intervertebral disk. As the annulas fibrosis ages it begins to lose the ability to contain the nucleus pulposus. This can cause the nucleus pulposus to herniate through the annulus fibrosis and apply pressure to the spinal cord or nerves branching from it. This condition is known as a prolapsed intervertebral disc, herniated disc or more commonly, a slipped disc. It is more prevalent in middle age and over but is in no way limited to these age groups.

There are two simple tests which can be performed to aid in diagnosis of this. One such method includes a straight leg raise. Here the individual lies on his or her back whilst the examiner places one hand at the base of the spine and the other under the ankle. As the leg is lifted the individual will experience pain in the back of the leg rather than the spine if a prolapsed intervertebral disc is present. The other test that can be performed is called 'Kerns sign'. While the individual is on his or her back, the examiner places one hand under the ankle and one over the knee. The knee and thigh are flexed to 90 degrees. The leg is then straightened. If on straightening a resistance is felt, there is a loss of ankle and knee jerk, and the individual feels pain after the procedure, then a prolapsed intervertebral disc may also be indicated.

Other tests which can be performed include computerized tomograghy, magnetic resonance imagery scan, discography and X-ray. These and other techniques are explained in detail by Maher.[13]

Congenital problems include scoliosis, which is a curvature of the spine in the coronal plane (face on) and spina bifida, which describes conditions of the spine where the posterior vertebral arches are defective. For minor cases surgery may not be indicated, and it can be treated by exercising correctly and taking precautions. Corrective surgery will be necessary in more severe cases.

Spondylolysis is a break or defect in the neural arch between the superior and inferior articulating processes. This defect is composed of fibrocartilaginous tissue rather than bone. This condition may progress to spondylolisthesis if not treated promptly, usually with a support brace. Spondylolisthesis describes the forward subluxation (movement) of one vertebra on another. There are different reasons for this and, generally, surgery will be required.

Degenerative problems include osteoporosis and osteoarthritis:

- Osteoporosis involves a severe reduction in the skeletal bone mass. This can lead to deformity and fractures. Although most common in the hips, spinal fractures can occur, mainly in the lumbar region. Spinal deformity, loss of height and chronic back pain are three of the symptoms observed.
- Osteoarthritis can also cause long-term back pain due to its inflammatory nature. Care has to be taken, as the cervical spine especially is weakened by this disorder and fractures leading to paralysis or death can occur. When having surgery, a soft collar should be worn for support and the anaesthetist reminded to take care when tilting the head on intubation.

Nursing care for chronic back pain

Before we can hope to treat or help the individual with their pain it is essential for an accurate, in-depth assessment. This should include assessment of possible problems causing the pain as the treatments are varied. For example, the rigorous exercise used in ankylosing spondylitis (a condition where the vertebrae are fusing together) would cause even more pain and harm for someone with a prolapsed intervertebral disc.

An accurate assessment of the individual's pain is also necessary if effective care is to be commenced. What is the pain like? Is it sharp or like a dull throb? Is it localized in one area or over a large area?

Although clinicians ask patients to remember their past pain and how treatment helped, Feine[14] found that questioning alone does not provide an accurate assessment in cases of chronic pain. She found that remembered levels of pain were inaccurate and became more severe over time. The assessment of past pain was also affected by the level of pain at the time of questioning. Ratings of relief increased over time even if other measures such as pain scoring did not. Feine[14] recommends that, to assist in accurate assessment of pain over a long period, the use of a diary can be beneficial, where a scoring system assists in recording levels of pain over a given time. Accurate assessment of pain is essential for effective treatment and a better understanding can be gained from elsewhere in this book.

Education leads to knowledge, which leads to power[15]

The process of giving information, which empowers an individual, is needed when seeking to help patients with chronic back pain. The process of self-empowerment enables individuals to take more control over their lives, and should enable them to become more independent. Pellino and Oberst[16] investigated the link between perception of control over chronic low back pain and the level of pain reported. They found that those who perceived higher levels of personal control reported less pain than those who perceived no control. Davis[3] recognizes that promoting independence is a role nurses should undertake. Whilst in hospital, this outcome should be reflected in the planning of care.

A holistic approach will be needed in order for this to be achieved. With regard to chronic back pain, there are a number of issues that will be especially relevant. Once pain is effectively tackled it means that movement is easier. A positive self-image should be promoted, thereby reducing patient anxiety and helping to lead to an understanding of self-care. Any knowledge deficit should be met with education, so that the individual understands the relevant problems and how to overcome them. Impaired physical mobility should be addressed and ways sought to enable greater independence by maintaining optimum physical ability.

Cohen[17] discusses the use of a health care belief model in the treatment of those with chronic low back pain. This can be used as a framework when the aim is to self-empower an individual. She acknowledges important points; for example, even when no diagnosis is evident, an individual should never feel that their pain is not believed. We are reminded that the UKCC[18] code of professional conduct states it is the responsibility of all nurses to take any measure that will enhance the well-being of the patient.

Cohen[17] acknowledges that the health belief model does not meet the standards required by a theory, but believes it to be a useful tool when planning care. The model has been summarized by Sheeran and Abraham.[19] First, there is the individual's perception of threat related to a disease. Secondly, there is the consequence of one's behaviour towards the disease. This is viewed in terms of vulnerability, and the severity of the illness, balancing what is thought to be the benefits of behaviour that is health related with the cost or perceived problems of carrying out that behaviour. They suggest that the health belief model incorporates cues that may prompt an individual to act. These could be intrinsic or extrinsic.

A similar framework has been devised at the Walton Centre for Neurology and Neurosurgery in Liverpool by the Pain Research Institute. They have devised a ten-point plan, which they have shown helps six out of ten individuals with chronic back pain. All of the plan has to be followed or it will be ineffective. It states:

1 Accept you have pain.
2 Pace yourself.
3 Be as active as you can for your age.
4 Take time for relaxation.
5 Take your painkillers correctly.
6 Be aware of what makes your pain worse.
7 Do not let the pain get the upper hand.
8 Get everyone on your side.
9 Form a link with others.
10 Do not give up.

By using such an approach it is possible to plan care that enables the individual with chronic back pain to accept the pain, not to fear it, and to show them how decisions they make will affect their health and levels of pain. Many studies have shown that this empowerment has effectively reduced chronic back pain.[5,20,21]

Pain relief

Most individuals are looking for relief from pain when they present to their GP or hospital outpatient department. There are many aspects which need to be taken into account before medication can be prescribed; current medication being taken and a past history of drug abuse are but two of these. It should be explained to the patient that it may not be possible to fully alleviate the pain, but that the most effective analgesia will be sought.

Analgesia works in different ways: opioids, for example, act on the hypothalamus and work by the removal of the memory or subjective distress of pain. They do not block pain. This means if patients are asked whether they are comfortable they may reply 'Yes'. However, by asking whether they are in pain, or how much it hurts, you are 'reminding' them of the pain, or bringing it to their attention, so that they may well respond that it is painful. Other analgesics, such as paracetamol, block the pain message while in the nerve. In terms of the gate theory of pain, paracetamol is thought to block the gate so reducing the strength of the message.

Opioids such as morphine sulphate are commonly used in the treatment of chronic malignant pain, but it has been suggested they may have a place in treating chronic non-malignant pain. York and Paice[22] discuss the long-term use of opioids administered via an intraspinal pump, an idea first developed in the USA. This remains controversial. It is believed to be safe and effective, yet there remain reservations over the possibility of tolerance and addiction. Much research into chronic malignant pain has shown that these problems are rare if opioids are used appropriately. Portenoy[23] provides an overview of this subject.

Oral analgesia may vary in strength, the method by which it works and

the classification of the drug. As everyone is unique, different medications will suit different individuals, and it may be necessary to re-
evaluate effectiveness until the most suitable match is found.

Transcutaneous electrical nerve stimulation (TENS) machines give
electrical impulses from pads attached to the skin. This is thought to
interfere with messages carried in the Aδ and C fibres in sensory nerves.
This mechanism has not yet been proven, and exactly how it works is not
known. This method of pain relief can, however, be helpful to those with
chronic back pain and is discussed in greater detail in a subsequent
chapter. As TENS has no significant side-effects it has potential as a
form of analgesia, and its positive role as a placebo can also not be
ignored.[13]

Non-steroidal anti-inflammatory drugs (NSAIDs) can be used if
precautions are taken to avoid gastrointestinal irritation that can result
from prolonged use. For example, the individual needs to be educated to
take NSAIDs with food. They are used in preference to steroidal anti-
inflammatories due to the number of side-effects steroids have in
prolonged use. NSAIDs work by reducing inflammation. This can aid
mobility and, as pressure is reduced on nerves, can also reduce levels of
pain. Pain is further reduced as NSAIDs inhibit bradykinin release, which
is known to activate the pain receptors. As with other medication,
different NSAIDs will suit different individuals, and alternatives may
need to be tried.

Lumbar epidurals have successfully been used in the treatment of
lower back pain where open surgery is considered unnecessary or
undesirable. They usually consist of a local anaesthetic and a steroid.
Although they can be very effective, lumbar epidurals can take up to 6
weeks to be fully effective, and the patient should be aware that relief will
not be instantaneous. The patient should also be aware before the
procedure of the risk, however slight, of damage to the spinal cord. This
could result in more pain or even paralysis.

Tricyclic antidepressants have been used, in low-dose form, effectively
in many cases of chronic pain. Their effectiveness in long-term back pain
appears to be limited to individuals who have an associated major
depression and who require antidepressant doses.[24]

Corsets and braces are used to give support, usually to the lumbar
spine. Collars can also be used to support the cervical spine in those with
neck pain. They range in design from material/foam for the neck,
providing light support, to ridged plastic corsets, which almost fully
restrict the spine. Corsets are mainly used after surgery, but are also
beneficial in conservative treatment as they allow the spine support and
restrict movement identified as high risk, such as twisting and bending.[25]
This gives the affected area a chance to rest and heal.

Positioning of the body is still an underused method of pain control. As
nurses, we often are too focused on the giving of medication rather than
seeking a simpler alternative, which can be just as effective. The
individual needs education on correct posture when sitting, walking and
lifting. 'Twenty-four hour back care' is a phrase becoming more prevalent
within nursing. This should be applied to everyone, especially those who
have long-term back pain, and can have a significant effect.

The use of heat and cold pads may be of benefit to some individuals. The pad can be placed onto the affected area or, if this is too painful, onto an area near the site, acupuncture points or along the nerve route between the site of pain and the brain. Care needs to be taken that the temperatures used are not too extreme and do not cause pain on application. They should not be used on those who have vascular problems, recent surgery on or near where the pad is to be placed, or where there is an area of recent swelling. Cold pads should not be used near the stomach if there is a past history of ulcers as it increases gastric activity.

When in bed, bending the knees by 30 degrees reduces pressure on the spinal cord, thereby reducing pain. Teaching the patient how to 'log roll' also eases pain and encourages better posture. It involves the individual being turned, ensuring the spine is moved as one combined unit without allowing any twisting of the body. In an acute setting after injury or surgery this should not be attempted unless a nurse trained in this procedure is present otherwise serious injury could occur.

Bed rest is often recommended for treatment of back pain. Twenty-three out of 24 hours is recommended for best effect, the other hour being set aside for hygiene needs.[25] This should be tried for a period of about 3–4 weeks before benefit is assessed. It should be remembered that if someone has been lying flat for some time, the blood pressure adapts to the prone position and, therefore, when the individual gets out of bed suddenly, the pressure is not sufficient to perfuse the brain. This can cause dizziness and a fainting episode.

Relaxation techniques, especially the use of imagery, have been successfully used in the treatment of chronic back pain. The individual, with help at first, will be guided to think of a scene or image which for them is relaxing. This may be a deserted tropical beach or gentle mountain stream. Whatever the focus, this method has the benefit of distracting from the pain with no side-effects, and is discussed in more detail in Chapter 12.

There are also alternative therapies available. These include aromatherapy, reflexology and hypnotism. Although not often available under the NHS, some find them beneficial when in chronic pain and prefer their use to taking medication for long periods of time. Hypnotism is discussed in Chapter 12.

Education

As discussed earlier, education is needed for those with chronic back pain. Not only does it enable them to develop an internal locus of control (they feel in control rather than others exerting control over them), but it also aids in reducing pain and preventing further injury.

General tips that can be given include being aware of extra body weight, as this will cause more strain on the spine. Smoking reduces the blood and nutrient supply to the discs, as nicotine is a vasoconstrictor. Keeping active within known limitations and not staying on bed rest for more than 48 hours, unless advised by medical staff, will help prevent the back from stiffening up.

Posture is important when standing as well as sitting. When standing and bending forwards to 90 degrees, with no load in hand, the human spine is under tremendous pressure (up to five times its load when standing erect) and is at serious risk of injury. Standing upright encourages the natural curves of the spine to support the body with the least strain. Activities that involve standing often promote asymmetrical postures. This can often be alleviated by placing one leg on a small platform. For example, when ironing, one can rest a foot on the Yellow Pages or telephone directory. When washing up, one can open the cupboard door below the sink and rest a foot on the bottom shelf.

When sitting, the same pressure is placed on the spine as bending to 90 degrees when standing. The back should be well supported to help keep its natural shape. Preferably, the chair should have arm supports to prevent the arms resting forwards and taking the spine out of alignment. The same principle applies to sitting in a car. Back pain sufferers should be told that, when getting in, they should turn to face away from the car. With one hand on the door frame and the other on the top of the seat, they should gently lower themselves into the car, moving the body as one unit (i.e. no bending). The legs should be swung into the car to avoid a twisting motion. The car seat can be tilted back to spread weight through the spine when going over bumps in the road. Travellers should take frequent stops and, at the end of the trip, should not lift anything until the stiffness from the journey has eased.

Low level activities, such as emptying the washing machine, encourage spinal flexion or stooping. This can be overcome by crouching down and separating the task into two movements. To reduce the load on the spine when making the bed one can kneel on the floor.

When resting or sleeping in bed it is important to ensure that the bed is not too soft or hard, as both cause the spine to move out of alignment and will increase stress placed on the back, as well as pain. Getting out of bed can involve much bending and twisting. The individual needs education on a low-risk method. If they are to get out of bed on the left, they need to roll onto their left side, positioning themselves on the edge of the bed. They then flex at the knee and hip to 90 degrees so the calf and feet are just over the side of the bed. By pushing up with the right hand, keeping the back straight and allowing the weight of the legs to help, they can sit on the side of the bed ready to stand. Personal experience has shown this method to be almost pain-free when suffering severe back pain on movement.

When washing, a shower causes less strain than a bath. If only a bath is available then kneeling rather than sitting should be tried, with a non-slip mat. When drying feet, sitting minimizes the bending necessary. If difficulty is experienced when dressing it can be overcome by lying on the bed and bending the knees to put on trousers, socks and so on. In this way, more movement is possible, with less pain, as there is less strain on the spine.

During lifting there will always be stress to the spine. This cannot be removed entirely, but there are ten guidelines which will help to reduce it.

1 Know your limitations.
2 Plan your lift; ask for help if needed.
3 Keep your back straight when lifting.
4 Position feet to give a stable base.
5 Do not use back muscles when lifting, use the leg muscles.
6 Brace stomach muscles, to support the spine.
7 Do not twist when lifting, move your feet.
8 Keep the load close to your body when lifting.
9 Move at a normal speed; moving quickly may lead to other guidelines being disregarded, while moving too slowly increases the time for which the back is supporting the load.
10 When carrying loads, anything which can be divided should be done symmetrically so that the weight is carried evenly and the spine is not disaligned.

Activity and exercise should be encouraged, as this helps to reduce the episodes of back pain and aids quicker recovery. Any exercises that increase back pain or leg pain should not be continued. With this in mind, beneficial exercises include, in particular, swimming. However, if breast-stroke is not performed correctly it may increase back pain, so that the stroke should be changed. Walking is another good exercise, but rest is required if pain begins to increase. Some individuals find benefit from aerobics if twisting and strenuous bending exercises are avoided, and others benefit from weight training. Great care with technique needs to be taken, and these activities need to be stopped immediately if pain increases. Jogging is not recommended as it involves jolting the spine.

Specific back exercises can be taught to help improve flexibility. Movement is affected by back pain as muscle groups around the spine tend to tighten. Exercises include specific leg stretches and pelvic tilting. These are best taught by a physiotherapist or back-care specialist nurse.

Conclusion

Chronic back pain is a condition that is becoming more common and is something with which the individual has to live day after day. Nurses need to be aware of how to help empower the individual, thereby assisting them in coming to terms with their pain and taking an active role in its treatment.

Different methods of pain relief need to be tried and assessed, with the most suitable being chosen. By giving education on back care and exercises, the individual feels involved in treatment. This allows them to feel a valued member of the team, and they are more likely to comply with the plan of care as a result.

As there are many treatments available and many causes and types of pain, a multidisciplinary team approach for chronic back pain is needed. The nurse will need to work closely with the other members of the team and the individual, acting as advocate when necessary. Nursing practice needs to be based on an accurate knowledge of the condition causing the problem, if known. At all times the individual should be believed if they say they are in pain, or the beneficial effects of communication between the individual and nurse will cease.

This chapter has explored the cost of chronic back pain, to both society and the individual, and in both social and economic terms. The nurse should be aware that the individual has had back pain for at least three months and in many cases longer. They may have seen numerous specialists and been given conflicting advice. They may feel that their pain is not believed. If the nurse is to develop a rapport, she needs to be prepared to listen and to believe what she is told. This relationship, based on trust, is the foundation for the nurse when planning holistic care, working with the individual towards reducing or alleviating their chronic back pain.

Summary
- Back pain costs the United Kingdom a considerable amount of money each year.
- Causes may either be mechanical or inflammatory.
- Correct diagnosis is essential before commencement of treatment.
- For those in pain, self-empowerment is an essential process in gaining control over the pain.
- There are useful frameworks to use in the treatment of chronic pain.
- The correct analgesia for the individual needs to be selected.
- There are other methods of pain relief as well as drug therapy.

References

1. McCaffrey, M. (1983) *Nursing the Patient in Pain*. Cambridge: Harper and Row.
2. Agency for Health Care Policy and Research. (1995) Acute low back problems in adults: assessment and treatment. *Orthopaedic Nursing*, 14(5), 37–52.
3. Davis, P. (1997) Pain when we move. *Journal of Orthopaedic Nursing*, 1, 147–53.
4. Bonica, J. (1990) *The Management of Pain*, 2nd edn. Philadelphia: Lea and Febiger.
5. Chase, J. (1992) Outpatient management of low back pain. *Orthopaedic Nursing*, 11(1), 11–20.
6. Office of Health Economics (1985) *Back Pain*. London: HMSO.
7. Waddle, G. (1996). Low back pain: a twentieth century healthcare enigma. *Spine*, 21, 2820–5.
8. Linton, S. (1998) The socioeconomic impact of chronic back pain: is anyone benefiting? *Pain*, 75, 163–5.
9. Bellamy, R. (1997) Compensation neurosis. *Clinical Orthopaedics and Related Research*, 336, 94–106.
10. Braggins, S. (1994) *The Back: Functions, Malfunctions and Care*. London: Mosby.
11. Tortora, G. and Grabowski, S. (1996) *Principles of Anatomy and Physiology*. Cambridge: Harper and Row.
12. Brooker, C. (1998) *Human Structure and Function*. London: Mosby International.
13. Maher, A., Salmond, S. and Pellino, T. (1994) *Orthopaedic Nursing*. Philadelphia: W. B. Saunders.
14. Feine, J., Lavigne, G., Dao, T. *et al.* (1998) Memories of chronic pain and perceptions of relief. *Pain*, 77, 137–41.
15. Blanchard, D. (1990) What women can do to protect against osteoporosis. *Registered Nurse*, October, pp. 60–4.

16. Pellino, T. and Oberst, M. (1992) Perceptions of control and appraisal of illness in chronic low back pain. *Orthopaedic Nursing*, 11(1), 22–6.
17. Cohen, S. (1997) Using a health belief model to promote increased wellbeing in obese patients with chronic low back pain. *Journal of Orthopaedic Nursing*, 1, 89–93.
18. United Kingdom Central Council for Nursing, Midwifery and Health Visiting (1992) *Code of Professional Conduct*, 3rd edn. London: UKCC.
19. Sheeran, P. and Abraham, C. (1996) The health belief model. In: Conner, M. and Norman, P. (eds), *Predicting Health Behaviour*. Buckingham: Open University Press.
20. Erskine, A. and de C Williams, A. C. (1989) Chronic pain. In: Broom, A. (ed.), *Health Psychology: Process and Applications*. London: Chapman and Hall.
21. Rosenstock, I., Strecher, V. and Becker, M. (1988) Social learning theory and the health belief model. *Health Education Quarterly*, 15(2), 175–83.
22. York, M. and Paice, J. (1998) Treatment of low back pain with intraspinal opioids delivered via implanted pumps. *Orthopaedic Nursing*, May/June, 61–8.
23. Portenoy, R. (1994) Opioid therapy for chronic nonmalignant pain: current status. In: Feilds, H. and Leibeskind, J. (eds), *Progress in Pain Research and Management*. Seattle, WA: IASP Press.
24. Atkinson, J. (1989) Psychopharmacologic agents in the treatment of pain syndromes. In: Tollison, C. (ed.), *Handbook of Chronic Pain Management*. London: Williams and Wilkins.
25. Scott, J. (1994) Spinal problems. In: Davis, P. (ed.), *Nursing the Orthopaedic Patient*. Edinburgh: Churchill Livingstone.

7

Malignant pain: management

K. Penn and C. Duncombe

Introduction

Pain is a more terrible lord of mankind than even death himself.[1]

This chapter will define the term palliative in the context of managing malignant or cancer pain, so that the reader may show an appreciation of the principles of pain control and demonstrate how they guide management. The use, place, limitations and misconceptions associated with strong opioids will be described, so that the reader may better understand the relevance and appropriateness of both pharmacological and non-pharmacological interventions.

The term palliative in the context of palliative care has been defined to be 'the active total care of patients whose disease is no longer responsive to curative treatment' integrating the physical, psychological, social, spiritual and cultural aspects of care for patients and their families.[2] Clearly this cohesive, broad approach can be applied to many specialties and, indeed, is a desirable objective of care in many situations. The distinction between generic and specialist palliative care has therefore arisen, the latter being applied to those 'professionally trained staff with recognized post-qualification specialist training and clinical experience in palliative care services'.[3]

In keeping with the World Health Organization definition some pictorial models perceive the illness trajectory along a linear scale with the introduction of specialist palliative care at a time when all avenues of active/curative treatment have been exhausted (Figure 7.1). Not surprisingly, this has engendered a negative image, with palliative care being viewed as only appropriate at a time when 'nothing more can be done' in terms of manipulating the disease process. Other models recognize that a palliative approach can be relevant and appropriate from the moment of diagnosis, with the palliative contribution increasing as

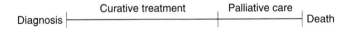

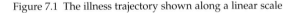

Figure 7.1 The illness trajectory shown along a linear scale

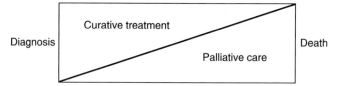

Figure 7.2 The palliative contribution increasing as illness and associated symptoms progress

illness and associated symptoms progress, complementing the work of other specialties also involved in the care of the patient (Figures 7.2 and 7.3). These models recognize the importance of intervention being according to clinical need, not diagnosis or stage of disease alone. Obviously the appropriateness of any intervention will vary between individuals and, in any one individual, it varies over time.

The fluctuating interface between curative and palliative approaches depicted in Figure 7.3 is how palliation should be viewed in the context of this chapter. Palliative management of malignant pain, therefore, refers globally to those interventions aimed at mitigating cancer-related pain at any stage of the disease process, and which may draw on the expertise of many professionals at various time points. The emphasis is on clinical need and need not be driven by the stage of disease process.

The earlier chapter on chronic malignant pain has explored in depth the scale and complexity of cancer pain, but it is worth revisiting some of the points raised. Pain is a multifaceted phenomenon. The focus for this chapter is management approaches that aim to modulate the physical experience of pain. It is vital not to lose sight of those other components that affect the patient's reaction to this symptom, namely the spiritual, psychological, social and cultural. In addition, we as nurses must not underestimate the extent of the problem and, moreover, our contribution in dealing with it. In 1992 60% of deaths from cancer occurred in hospital.[4] Considering that pain is present at diagnosis in one-third of cases, increasing to two-thirds in advanced cancer, the extent of the problem is revealed. Rather alarmingly, however, it would appear that despite advances in our understanding of the symptom and the array of methods available to relieve pain there has been little change in the number of patients – in excess of 80% – reporting the symptom between 1969 and 1987.[5,6] Having highlighted this, it is still important to maintain a sense of perspective when caring for this group of patients. It is all too

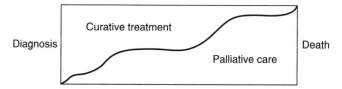

Figure 7.3 The fluctuating interface between curative and palliative approaches

easy to become blinkered and to assume that every pain is directly or indirectly caused by the cancer itself. Considering that cancer principally affects an elderly population, other pre-existing or new painful conditions may well arise related to other non-malignant pathology such as osteoarthritis.

This chapter will not portray management in a prescriptive or didactic format. The intention is to marry the factual basis of the topic with those real world issues presented to us within the acute hospital setting. Theory and clinical practice will therefore be combined. In-depth analysis of those principles that guide pain management will initially be discussed, moving on to discuss the role of analgesics and co-analgesics. At this point, with the exception of morphine, only broad classifications of drugs will be considered. A fundamental understanding is required of the basics before considering more specific areas of drug therapy. Readers are therefore directed to other specialist sources for more information. A recurring theme will be the importance of a multi- and interdisciplinary approach. Those interventions not considered elsewhere in this book and which will be covered in this chapter include radiotherapy and chemotherapy.

Principles of pain management

General principles

Comprehensive and repeated assessment, including physical examination, underpins successful pain management. This is no task to be taken lightly and, moreover, is not a single event. Throughout the literature the term 'assessment' is consistently written in the singular and may account for the failure to see this task as a continuous activity. It need not involve the completion of comprehensive pain charts but must not simply be a cursory enquiry 'Do you have any pain?' at the time of the drug round. A detailed history must be taken, preferably directly from the patient, examining the site(s) of pain, onset, diurnal variables, subjective descriptors and those factors which exacerbate/ameliorate the pain. At this stage knowledge of current medication and its effectiveness is invaluable as it may avoid waste, both in terms of time and resources.

> Derek, aged 63, had severe rib pain secondary to metastatic bone disease arising from primary prostatic malignancy. On admission he was prescribed paracetamol 1 g every 6 hours and sustained release diclofenac, yet at home full dose weak opioids in combination with a non-steroidal anti-inflammatory drug had been ineffective.

It has been said that 'the general hospital as a setting for terminal care has disturbing deficiencies'.[7] Certainly, from the above example it would appear that basic principles are not adhered to, and yet considering the scale of the problem, discussed earlier, our approach should be consistent, logical and accurate. More recently, the research of Bruster[8] uncovered discrepancies in the management of pain, not specifically applied to cancer patients. A total of 5150 randomly selected NHS patients who had recently been discharged from hospital were surveyed on all aspects of their care: 86% responded to the interview questionnaire. Patients were generally highly satisfied with the care they received, but specific areas of care, such as pain management, received criticism. Sixty-one per cent of patients suffered pain during their admission, with 87% of those rating it to be severe or moderate. Analgesics had to be requested in 42% of patients experiencing pain, and failed to be administered immediately in 41%.

Identifying the quality of the pain, as defined by the patient, can assist the assessor to determine the type of pain and its likely response to different interventions; for example, descriptors such as shooting, burning and stabbing tend to indicate neuropathic pain, whereas dull and aching can be applied to bone pain. For some patients, however, the requirement to describe their pain by assigning descriptors is too difficult. We, as health care professionals, must be careful not to impose our own expectations which may leave patients feeling responsible when therapy is unsuccessful.

The causes of cancer pain include tumour infiltration of pain sensitive structures and injury to nerves, bone and soft tissue as a result of anti-cancer therapy. Broadly, pain may be distinguished as either somatic, visceral or neuropathic. Somatic pain refers to the activation of nociceptors in cutaneous and deep tissues such as bone. It is characterized by aching or gnawing sensations, and is usually well localized. Visceral pain is poorly localized and applies to thoracic and abdominal viscera which have been infiltrated, compressed or stretched secondary to primary or metastatic disease. Neuropathic pain describes damage to peripheral and/or central nerve structures, either as a consequence of tumour infiltration or compression or treatment with surgery, chemotherapy and/or radiotherapy.[9] The manifestation of neuropathic pain is frequently severe and presents many challenges to the managing team, not least because of its limited response to opioid therapy.

The approaches to management include modification of the disease process, elevation of the pain threshold by pharmacological and non-pharmacological means, interruption of the nerve pathways and modification of lifestyle and environment. This can only be achieved successfully by involving a wide range of expertise and adopting a multi- and interdisciplinary approach.

Where possible, relevant clinical investigations are important to diagnose the source of the pain and to guide management. For example, a suspected pathological fracture can be easily confirmed by X-ray and subsequent pain relief achieved with surgery. Obviously, the potential benefits of investigating and subsequently intervening must be weighed against the potential risks and trauma incurred to the patient.

Patient, family and professional expectations

The importance of thorough and ongoing physical assessment has been addressed but, in order to construct a complete picture of the pain's

impact on the patient's and family's lifestyles, assessment of psychological, spiritual and social aspects are equally important. This can be
achieved by asking questions such as:

'What does the pain mean to you?'
'How are you coping with it?'
'How is it affecting you in your day-to day-life/ your relationship
with others?'

Establishing a wide perspective on these issues will inform the next
stage: goal-setting. At first glance it may not be unreasonable to assume
that this is an unnecessary, time-wasting exercise, as the complete
resolution of pain would be the desired objective in every situation.
However, this is where our own professional expectations need to be
reconciled with those of the patient and the family. In some circumstances
patients will aim for partial pain relief. It is not unusual for patients to use
the presence of mild, residual pain to monitor disease progression.

Immediately the relevance of psychological support is realized, as an
increase in the level of pain or the manifestation of a new pain can
obviously leave patients feeling frightened and distressed. A consistent
objective of pain management should, therefore, be accurate diagnosis of
the cause. Unfortunately, this may not always be possible. Where
complete relief from pain is the desired objective, goals should be
achievable, and also achievable within a clear time-frame. A three-step
approach is frequently adopted, aiming first for relief of pain at night,
secondly at rest and thirdly on movement. The nurse's role in providing
clear and consistent information and explanation cannot be overstated.
Seeking the patient's involvement and cooperation in pain management
will reduce fear and anxiety, frequently associated with lack of
knowledge, and enhance patient and family confidence.

Principles applied to the administration of analgesics

Most cancer pain is relieved with orally administered analgesics, either
alone or in combination with adjuvant (co-analgesic) drug therapy. An
understanding of those terms frequently applied to analgesics is
essential, namely opiate, opioid and co-analgesic. Opiate refers to those
drugs, natural and semisynthetic, derived from the juice of the opium
poppy (e.g. morphine). Opioid is a general term describing those drugs
with morphine-like activity, their effects being activated by binding to
opioid receptors and antagonized by naloxone (e.g. diamorphine).[10] A co-
analgesic has been defined to be 'a drug that has a primary indication
other than pain but is analgesic in some painful conditions'[11] (e.g.
antidepressants, anticonvulsants, corticosteroids).

It is fundamentally important to tailor analgesic therapy to the needs
of the individual patient by selecting the most appropriate analgesic
and/or co-analgesic, administered in the right dose and at the right time.
Adherence to these principles will maximize pain relief and minimize
adverse effects.

A logical, three-step approach to managing cancer-related pain is illustrated in Figure 7.4, which presents the World Health Organization's 'analgesic ladder'.[2] The principles governing the use of this tool are that persistent or increasing pain requires a move up the ladder to step two, and so on, rather than switching medication for an alternative drug of similar efficacy. Regular administration of the analgesic is a vital component of this approach as the pain is almost always, by definition, ongoing. Health care professionals therefore need a good understanding of the dosing intervals of drugs and patients may need clear explanations of the rationale for regular administration. A most useful aide-mémoire to summarize these points is reflected in the following phrase:

(a) By mouth
(b) By the clock
(c) By the ladder

Step 1 includes those non-opioid analgesics, such as paracetamol and aspirin +/− adjuvant, progressing at step 2 to a weak opioid such as codeine in addition to paracetamol +/− adjuvant, and at step 3 the weak opioid is substituted for a strong opioid such as morphine. These guidelines are accepted steps that are known to relieve pain in clinical practice. It is important to note, however, that there is much that remains unknown about precise mechanisms of pain pathways and actions of analgesia.

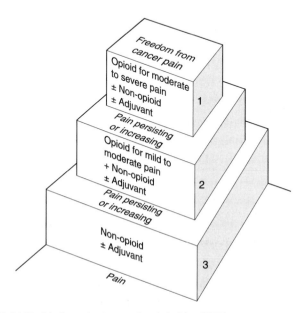

Figure 7.4 World Health Organization analgesic ladder (1990)

Non-opioid drugs

Paracetamol and non-steroidal anti-inflammatory drugs (NSAIDs) are the most commonly used non-opioid drugs in cancer pain management.[12]

NB: In some palliative care texts NSAIDs are classified as co-analgesics, with only aspirin being included in non-opioid drugs.

Paracetamol is clinically established as an effective analgesic for mild pain, although its mode(s) of action are not clearly understood. It can also be very useful at steps 2 and 3 of the analgesic ladder to complement weak and strong opioid action. Apart from the well-known problems of over-dosage and caution in the presence of hepatic damage/failure, its relative side-effect-free profile renders it a particularly effective drug for pain management at all levels.

Commonly used NSAIDs include aspirin, ibuprofen, naproxen and diclofenac. It is recommended in palliative care to use NSAIDs that have a shorter half-life to enable rapid assessment of efficacy followed by faster dose increase if needed.[12] In addition, the efficacy and known toxicity of individual NSAIDs needs to be taken into account. For example, the side-effect profile of ibuprofen is less, but so is the analgesic effect; aspirin at full therapeutic dose is effective but gives a high incidence of gastrointestinal side-effects. For these reasons, among others, it is suggested that diclofenac and naproxen are two of the best NSAIDs to consider initially in this patient population. Indomethacin is a useful back-up as it is more potent but also more toxic.[12]

Opioids

The management of cancer pain commonly requires the use of opioid drugs.[13] It is helpful to understand something of their mechanism of action, and hence their side-effects.

Opioids are agonists of at least three receptor sites sited in the brain and spinal cord, μ, κ and δ. The responses mediated by activating these receptor sites include not only analgesia but also the adverse effects commonly encountered with this group of drugs, including nausea, vomiting, respiratory depression and constipation.[14]

Weak opioids

Weak opioids constitute step 2 of the WHO analgesic ladder. Codeine is the standard weak opioid analgesic, either used alone or in varying strengths and combinations with non-opioids. Dextropropoxyphene, in combination with paracetamol, is another common and useful drug for moderate pain.

Although, in general, it is not recommended to try another analgesic on the same 'step' of the ladder when pain is not controlled, weak opioids may be an exception because of the very low doses of codeine in some compound preparations. For example, co-codamol 8/500 contains 8 mg of codeine per tablet, co-dydramol 10 mg. If pain is not controlled on these lower doses, it can be beneficial to try the higher dose co-codamol 30/500 (30 mg codeine), codeine itself or dihydrocodeine before moving on to strong opioids. This decision will need to be balanced against the severity and nature of the pain in each individual.

In situations where the patient has been taking regular weak opioids and the pain remains uncontrolled, the conversion dose to strong opioids needs to be considered. It is generally held that oral weak opioids are approximately one-tenth of the strength of oral morphine and therefore the usual starting dose of oral morphine is 10 mg 4-hourly.[13]

More recently, advances in analgesic therapy have given rise to new drugs that are not included in the classic analgesic ladder. Tramadol is one such drug which is now thought to fit into the weak opioid category.[13] Currently, it is not commonly used in cancer pain management in the acute hospital setting.

Co-analgesics

As with non-opioids, co-analgesics can be used at all stages of the analgesic ladder where their use is indicated. Specialist palliative care advice may be helpful in these situations. It is worth noting that in some palliative care texts this group of drugs is termed adjuvant analgesics. The main groups classified under this heading are antidepressants, anticonvulsants and corticosteroids.[13]

Antidepressants (in particular the tricyclic group, e.g. amitriptyline, dothiepin) can be helpful in nerve injury/compression pain. It is proposed that their mode(s) of action include blocking chemicals in the nerve pathways. This type of pain is often described as shooting or burning and is classically only partially helped by morphine. In our experience, it can be helpful to start at a low dose (e.g. amitriptyline 10 mg nocté), particularly in the elderly, to minimize the impact of side-effects. The dose can then be increased according to pain response and side-effect tolerance. Typical side-effects of tricyclic antidepressants are mainly cardiovascular, with hypotension and arrythmias being the most serious, but also sedation and anti-cholinergic effects such as dry mouth, constipation and blurred vision. Two other points are worth highlighting: First, the full effect of this therapy may take up to 3 weeks to be established, although changes in the pain are often felt before then. Secondly, the patient will need a clear explanation of the rationale for using antidepressants as a co-analgesic rather than treatment for a psychological or psychiatric condition.

Similarly, anticonvulsants can be effective in treating nerve pain, it is thought by reducing nerve excitability. Carbamazepine and sodium valproate are probably the most commonly used. It has been suggested that this class of co-analgesic is better at relieving shooting/paroxysmal nerve pain, however there is debate about this and, on current evidence, there is probably little difference between anticonvulsants and anti-depressants.[13] Side-effects include sedation, dizziness, nausea and unsteadiness, which often improve over time.

Corticosteroids are used as co-analgesics in malignant pain caused by nerve compression, liver capsule pain and bone involvement. It is thought that their mode(s) of action include reducing peri-tumour oedema. The adverse effects of steroids are well known and need to be weighed up for each patient.

Other drugs classified as co-analgesics include anti-arrhythmics, the anaesthetic drug ketamine, muscle relaxants and antihistamines. Specialist advice should be sought where pain is unresponsive to the more common analgesics and co-analgesics.

The use of co-analgesics can add to the burden of illness for the patient, both in terms of more tablets to take and side-effects to endure. It is, therefore, particularly important to assess their effectiveness and be prepared to stop them if the pain does not respond within the appropriate time scale, or side-effects become intolerable.

Strong opioids

Morphine

While, more recently, there have been important developments in the availability and administration of strong opioid analgesia, morphine remains the gold standard by which to titrate dose against effect. It is only by having a sound practical understanding of this drug that many of the fears and misconceptions held by staff will be dispelled.

Morphine metabolism occurs primarily in the liver, with approximately 90% being converted to metabolites, of which the largest component is the glucuronides.[14] They are significant because they ensure morphine is water soluble and, therefore, enable the drug to be excreted through the kidney.[14] The use of morphine in the presence of renal impairment, indicated by raised levels of serum creatinine, requires judicious consideration as the potential accumulation of morphine metabolites secondary to a reduced glomerular filtration rate increases the likelihood of undesirable, adverse effects. However, this alone is not a contraindication to its use. In our experience, extending the dosing interval to 6/8-hourly, to enable greater excretion of the metabolites, +/− reducing the dose, can avoid toxicity.

Many fears and misunderstandings prevail concerning the use of morphine and are held not only by the general public but also by health care professionals. The most common misunderstanding is that those problems encountered with the abuse of strong opioids are also met when they are used therapeutically. The fears of sedation, addiction and respiratory depression have all too frequently resulted in therapeutic underdosing, or the failure to prescribe them at all. Sadly, patients and their families often associate the introduction of morphine with the terminal phase of the disease process. Perhaps such opinion stems from our own prejudices as health care professionals. On how many occasions have you heard the death of a patient being attributed to the last dose of morphine?

Contrary to public belief, morphine can be safely used, if indicated, at any stage of disease and continued for many months. Difficulties are rarely encountered when reducing the dose or stopping treatment if the pain subsides following specific interventions (e.g. nerve blocks, chemotherapy, surgery and radiotherapy).

In order to achieve optimum pain control while minimizing undesirable adverse effects patients should be prescribed immediate release morphine with the same dose on an as-required basis for breakthrough pain, which may be given as often as required. For patients previously stabilized on regular doses of weak opioids the usual starting dose is 10 mg every 4 hours. Exceptions to this may apply if the patient is elderly and/or pre-existing renal problems are present. The total daily dose should be reviewed every 24 hours with adjustments taking account of the number of p.r.n. doses required in the previous 24 hours. As a general guide, titration usually occurs in increments of between 30 and 50%. Therefore, patients requiring a dose increase from 10 mg 4-hourly would progress to 15 mg, 20 mg, 30 mg, 40 mg, 60 mg etc. Once a stable 4-hourly dose has been reached, conversion to a longer-acting preparation can then take place. The total 24-hourly dose of morphine is calculated and this dose either divided by two for the 12-hourly preparations (e.g. MST) or left in total for the once-daily preparations now available.

Occasionally, 4-hourly administration of strong opioids may place an unreasonable burden on staff and patients, resulting in delays of administration. If this is the case, whilst not ideal, it may be possible to start treatment with a longer-acting morphine preparation, as described above. It is important to remember, however, that any side-effects or intolerance will take a correspondingly long time to remit.

As part of the ongoing assessment process the nurse's responsibility is to ascertain the effectiveness of the drug, coupled with careful monitoring of adverse effects. The initiation of morphine therapy does not guarantee pain relief. It is important to note that some pains are only partially morphine-responsive. These include nerve and bone pain in particular. Specific treatment for these is considered under 'co-analgesics'.

Signs of toxicity include confusion, visual hallucinations, pin-point pupils, respiratory depression and myoclonic jerking. In the presence of such symptoms the following questions need to be asked:

1 Is the pain morphine responsive?

Yes   reduce dose by 30–50%
Partly   reduce dose by 30–50% and consider adjuvant
         medication
No   reduce morphine administration by decreasing total dose
         by 30–50% every 24 hours.

2 Is renal failure/deteriorating renal function contributing to the presence of such symptoms?

Yes   consider extending dosing interval +/– reducing dose by
         30–50%

Other strong opioid preparations are available and used in palliative care, such as transdermal fentanyl, oxycodone, hydromorphone and methadone. These should be considered in conjunction with specialist advice.

Subcutaneous infusions are recommended only when the oral route is contraindicated, e.g. intractable vomiting, dysphagia, inability to swallow oral drugs due to weakness, and poor alimentary absorption. The drug commonly used is diamorphine, because of its high solubility, and which is three times more potent than oral morphine. The total 24 hour dose of oral morphine should therefore be calculated and divided by 3 to achieve the same analgesic effect.

Radiotherapy

Radiotherapy has an important role to play in the relief of cancer pain, particularly in the presence of bone metastases. Response rates have consistently been reported in the region of 80% with a significant proportion of patients reporting complete pain relief following either fractionated courses of 20–30 Gy over 1–2 weeks or a single dose of 8 Gy.[15] Such levels of pain relief are achieved up to 4 weeks from the time of treatment, during which time medication may need to be manipulated. Where patients are in hospital for at least some time following completion of treatment the nurse has a vital role in pain assessment, not only monitoring the effectiveness of treatment and the response to analgesia, but equally observing for any undesirable effects which may indicate that a dose reduction of analgesic or a step down the analgesic ladder is required. Even where treatment occurs in the outpatient setting the nurse should educate patients and their families about the expectations of treatment and forewarn them of the possibility that analgesia may need to be manipulated as treatment effects are noticed. Advice can therefore be sought promptly from the General Practitioner.

For patients whose skeletal disease is widespread, resulting in diffuse pain, wide-field or hemibody irradiation may be the treatment of choice. Interestingly, this method frequently results in pain relief within 24–48 hours, suggesting an alternative mechanism for analgesia compared with local irradiation. Unfortunately, greater toxicity accompanies such treatment. A period of bone marrow suppression is commonplace, and two-thirds of patients will experience gastrointestinal symptoms of nausea, vomiting or diarrhoea. Radiation pneumonitis is a rare but serious complication occasionally associated with upper hemibody irradiation.[15] More recently, the role of radioactive strontium in the management of pain caused by extensive skeletal disease has been realized; again this is a specialist procedure.[11]

The mechanism for modulating pain with radiotherapy is unclear. The obliteration of tumour cells undoubtedly occurs even after small, single doses of radiation, which results in pain relief. However, considering that pain relief is achieved up to several weeks following treatment with local irradiation compared with hours following widebody irradiation would suggest that other factors may also be important. Hoskin[15] suggests that local effects upon the host tissue, affecting osteoblast/osteoclast interaction and the release of pain-mediating agents, are equally important when it comes to achieving and maintaining pain relief.

The idea of radiotherapy is frequently a fearful concept for many patients and their families. The presence of large, heavy machinery, in addition to receiving treatment in isolation, often compounds one's vulnerability. Supporting patients in advance of treatment is an important nursing responsibility. Equally, the nurse should be aware of the site(s) to be treated and, working with the managing team, take any preventative measures which will minimize potential adverse effects; for example, where nausea may be an unpleasant side-effect, prophylactic anti-emetics will usually overcome this symptom. Where treatment is given as a fractionated course, patients require skin care advice, particularly where other factors may precipitate localized reaction. These include treatment to skin that is damaged or at risk of damage, for example previous surgery and pressure points, and areas of increased skin contact, i.e. skin folds. In addition, patients whose skin is sun-sensitive and who are receiving adjuvant treatment with radiosensitive chemotherapeutic agents are more susceptible.[16] Minimizing skin trauma is therefore essential and can only be achieved with presenting a clear educational message to patients and their families. Simple actions include:

- Keep area clean and dry, using pure unperfumed soap, and a patting rather than rubbing technique.
- Avoid metallic based talcum powders as this can lead to radiation scattering, in turn increasing dose to the skin.
- Avoid wet-shaving. Abrasions to radiated skin are slower to heal.
- Avoid wearing tight-fitting clothing and direct sunlight, both of which will cause unnecessary skin trauma.

Skin reactions often manifest themselves around 2–3 weeks following the start of treatment, explained by cell turnover in the epidermis.[17] In addition to prophylactic measures, monitoring skin integrity, both the entry and exit treatment sites, and taking action as necessary is an additional but no less important nursing responsibility.

Chemotherapy

Chemotherapy, or in this context cytotoxic drug administration, can be a useful symptom control agent but its use rests on the tumour's likely response plus a detailed assessment weighing up the potential risks against the presumed benefits.

The pain-relieving response mediated by cytotoxic drugs may not only depend on tumour regression but also may block cytokine release, a contributory factor in inflammation and the perception of pain.[18] Independent of tumour effect, these authors also consider that some analgesic effects are mediated by alterations to the peripheral and central neurotransmitter systems.

With reference to the work of Bonadonna and Molinari,[19] very good or complete pain relief has been achieved following cytotoxic drug treatment in the following primary cancers: breast, prostate, lymphomas, leukaemia and myeloma.

Non-pharmacological interventions

Elsewhere in this book the role of transcutaneous electrical nerve stimulation (TENS), massage, acupuncture and anaesthetic techniques will be discussed and explored in detail. To avoid repetition they are therefore not considered in this chapter, but this does not suggest that they are not significant management approaches in the treatment of malignant pain.

A wide range of methods are therefore available to us, but each needs to be considered on its own merits and within the context of clinical need. An individualized approach is therefore essential. Equally, an approach that depends on the unique contribution of a wide range of professional groups, drawing on their own areas of expertise while striving for a common goal will lead to optimal symptom control.

Conclusion

Rather than offering a prescriptive guide to the management of malignant pain, this chapter has explored those principles and techniques which contribute to the alleviation of this symptom. The factual basis of the topic has been combined with those real everyday issues which face us in the acute hospital setting and, where possible, solutions have been proposed. In this way we hope that we have avoided those divisions in theory and practice, so frequently referred to by clinicians and theorists alike.

The following case study brings to life many of the key points we wish to emphasize. To protect confidentiality, names have been changed.

Charlotte, aged 49, presented to palliative care specialists with severe, well-localized rectal pain, plus diffuse nerve pain affecting local nerve routes. She had been diagnosed with a malignant rectal tumour 2 years previously, the treatment for which comprised surgery, radiotherapy and chemotherapy. Faced with advanced local disease, and the responsibility of caring for two teenage children alone, she returned to family in England (South Africa had been her home for many years).

At presentation, she clearly described the level and characteristics of the pain and the impact this was having on her life, and her family's. She discussed the loss of her health and independence, and the resulting effects, in particular her perceived loss of identity as mother. Living in the knowledge of having incurable disease, pain served as a constant reminder of mortality; she openly feared for her children's welfare in the future.

Following detailed assessment and examination a combined approach using initially weak opioids, an NSAID plus antidepressants regime for the nerve pain was started. Little response was achieved. The addition of anticonvulsant therapy plus switching the weak opioids for morphine resulted in partial pain relief. Goals were renegotiated as to our and Charlotte's expectations of drug treatment alone; continuity of care in the community was achieved through regular communication with her GP. Involvement from physiotherapy and occupational therapy helped her to modify her lifestyle and to live within the constraints of her disease while referral to the social work department helped to ease the financial and social burden she perceived. Pain relief was achieved following the specialist intervention of the anaesthetists, who inserted an epidural.

Summary
- Pain is a multifaceted experience. As professionals we must not neglect the entire picture, paying equal attention to physical and psychosocial factors.
- Assessment and reassessment are key in the management cycle.
- Mutually acceptable goals between patient and professional should be set, and re-negotiated where necessary.
- Pharmacological management requires a logical, step-wise approach using both the analgesic ladder and, where necessary, adjuvant medication for specific indications.
- Involvement of the multidisciplinary team should accompany all stages of the management approach to be adopted. The level of involvement by any single professional must be according to clinical need.
- The nurse's responsibility for assessment, monitoring the response and side-effect profile of therapeutic modalities, communicating findings to those involved in the care of the patient and educating and supporting patients and their families cannot be overestimated.

Acknowledgements

We wish to acknowledge, with thanks, the contribution of our colleague and friend, Peter Pitcher for his assistance in writing this chapter.

References

1. Schweizer, A. (1947) *The Spiritual Life*. Boston: Beacon Press.
2. World Health Organization (1990) *Cancer Pain Relief and Palliative Care*. Geneva: WHO.
3. National Council for Hospice and Specialist Palliative Care Services (1995) *Specialist Palliative Care. A Statement of Definitions*. Occasional Paper 8. NCHSPCS.
4. Hospice Information Service (1996) *Hospice Facts and Figures*. Fact sheet 7. HIS.
5. Cartwright, A., Hockey, L. and Anderson, J. L. (1973) *Life before Death*. London: Routledge and Kegan Paul.
6. Seale, C. (1991) Death from cancer and death from other causes: the relevance of the hospice approach. *Palliative Medicine*, 5, 12–19.
7. Mount, B. M. (1976). The problem of caring for the dying in a general hospital; the palliative care unit as a possible solution. *CMA Journal*, 115, 119–21.
8. Bruster, S., Jarman, B., Bosanquet, N. *et al.* (1994) National survey of hospital patients. *British Medical Journal*, 309,1542–9.
9. Payne, R. and Gonzales, G. (1998) Pathophysiology of pain in cancer and other terminal diseases. In: Doyle, D., Hanks, G. W. C. and Macdonald, N. (eds), *Oxford Textbook of Palliative Medicine*, 2nd edn. Oxford: Oxford University Press, pp. 140–8.
10. Hanks, G. W., de Conno, F., Ripamonti, C. *et al.* (1996) Morphine in cancer pain: modes of administration. *British Medical Journal*, 312, 823–6.

11. Portenoy, R. K. (1998) Adjuvant analgesics in pain management. In: Doyle, D., Hanks, G. W. C. and Macdonald, N. (eds), *Oxford Textbook of Palliative Medicine*, 2nd edn. Oxford: Oxford University Press, pp. 187–203.

12. Rawlins, M. D. (1998) Non-opioid analgesics. In: Doyle, D., Hanks, G. W. C. and Macdonald, N. (eds), *Oxford Textbook of Palliative Medicine*, 2nd edn. Oxford: Oxford University Press, pp. 182–7.

13. Twycross, R. (1997) *Symptom Management in Advanced Cancer*, 2nd edn. Oxford: Radcliffe Medical Press.

14. Hanks, G. and Cherny, N. (1998) Opioid analgesic therapy. In: Doyle, D., Hanks, G. W. C. and Macdonald, N. (eds), *Oxford Textbook of Palliative Medicine*, 2nd edn. Oxford: Oxford University Press, pp. 331–55.

15. Hoskin, P.J. (1998) Radiotherapy in symptom management. In: Doyle, D., Hanks, G. W. C. and Macdonald, N. (eds), *Oxford Textbook of Palliative Medicine*, 2nd edn. Oxford: Oxford University Press, pp. 267–82.

16. Copp, K. (1989) Nursing patients having radiotherapy. In: Tiffany, R. and Borley, D. (eds), *Oncology for Nurses and Health Care Professionals*, 2nd edn, Volume 3: *Cancer Nursing*. London: Harper and Row, pp. 38–73.

17. Duchesne, G. and Horwich, A. (1989) The nature of radiotherapy. In: Tiffany, R. and Borley, D. (eds) *Oncology for Nurses and Health Care Professionals*, 2nd edn, Volume 1: *Pathology, Diagnosis and Treatment*. London: Harper and Row, pp. 223–45.

18. Osoba, D. and MacDonald, N. (1998) Principles governing the use of cancer chemotherapy in palliative care. In: Doyle, D., Hanks, G. W. C. and Macdonald, N. (eds), *Oxford Textbook of Palliative Medicine*, 2nd edn. Oxford: Oxford University Press, pp. 249–67.

19. Bonadonna, G. and Molinari, R. (1979) Role and limits of anticancer drugs in the treatment of advanced cancer pain. *Advances in Pain Research and Therapy*, 2, 131–44.

8
Pharmacology

M. Stuart Taylor

Introduction

The pharmacological control of pain should be considered as just one component in the amelioration of symptoms. Other chapters have given a background to the other elements such as the psychological aspects, physical methods of pain relief and nerve blocks.

By assessing the quality of pain, as well as its intensity, one can apply a structured approach to the analgesics used. The majority of chronic pain, whether associated with cancer or not, can be controlled with familiar drugs which can often be given by the oral route.

The WHO analgesic ladder[1] is often referred to when considering analgesics. In its original form it can sometimes be misunderstood. Very simply, 'non-opioid' drugs may be used with adjuvant drugs at any stage of the pain ladder. The only difference between grades of pain is the strength of the opioid used. Non-opioid drugs are sometimes taken to include anagelsics such as co-dydramol but, strictly speaking, these are weak opioids since they contain codeine. Adjuvant drugs include non-steroidal anti-inflammatory drugs (NSAIDs) and are listed below.

To explain the logic behind using different drugs together it is helpful to consider pain as the hub of a wheel. Many spokes radiate out from the hub, each of which represents a different mechanism for reducing pain. By using moderate doses of drugs with differing mechanisms of action one can create a synergistic effect of all drugs used – that is to say that

Table 8.1 Routes of delivery

Route	Abbreviation
Oral	o
Sublingual	sl
Rectal	pr
Subcutaneous	sc
Intramuscular	im
Intravenous	iv
Transcutaneous	tc

each type of drug enhances another type to a greater extent than if each were given alone.

Routes of delivery are shown in Table 8.1.

Non-opioids

Paracetamol

500–1000 mg q.d.s (to maximum 4 g/day) (o/pr)

NSAIDs   [note 1]

Diclofenac up to 150 mg/day (o/pr)   [note 2]
Ibuprofen up to 2.4 g/day (o)
Ketorolac 10 mg 4–6-hourly (o/im/iv)   [note 3]
Meloxicam 7.5–15 mg daily (o/pr)   [note 4]

Corticosteroids

See below under anti-emetic therapy.

Tricyclic antidepressants

Useful when burning, toothache component to pain; usually due to nerve involvement.

Amitriptyline – start at 10 mg nocté, increasing by 10 mg/night every 3 days to maximum of 100 mg nocté or until side-effects appear, such as dry mouth, sedation, blurred vision, constipation, urinary retention.

Anticonvulsant agents

Useful when stabbing, shooting component to pain.

Sodium valproate – 300 mg twice-daily, increasing by 200 mg/day at 3-day intervals to a maximum of 2.5 g/day in 2 divided doses.

Weak opioids

Co-dydramol

Dihydrocodeine 10 mg + Paracetamol 500 mg   [note 5]

Co-proxamol

Dextropropoxyphene 32.5 mg + Paracetamol 325 mg   [note 6]

Co-codamol

8/500 (Codeine 8 mg + Paracetamol 500 mg)
30/500 (Codeine 30 mg + Paracetamol 500 mg)   [note 7]

Dihydrocodeine (DF118)

30 mg 4-hourly   [note 8]

Notes

1. Avoid aspirin because of the significant risk of gastrointestinal bleeding with long-term use.
2. The im route should be avoided since it can cause cold abscess formation. It is worth considering the slow release (SR) formulation since the standard preparation only lasts approximately 4 hours for each dose.
3. May be used up to 90 mg daily via parenteral route but restrict use to 7 days. Limit dose in elderly to 40 mg/day by any route.
4. Currently considered to be one of the safest NSAIDs if concerned about effect on gut.
5. This can cause constipation, which should be treated early with appropriate laxatives.
6. This does not constipate, but the dextropropoxyphene can cause disturbing nightmares.
7. If one does not specify which strength of drug to use (i.e. 8/500 or 30/500) the weaker drug will be dispensed.
8. Constipation is minimized by using the lower dose of 30 mg as specified rather than 60 mg 6-hourly.

Strong opioids

Morphine

- Regular administration is vital because of the length of duration of immediate release morphine (4 hours).
- Reassure that morphine is generally not addictive whilst being taken for pain.
- Beware of side-effects when introducing morphine (see below).
- Start with a low dose and increase by 30–50% increments each day until pain comes under control or unless side-effects become a concern.

Immediate release

Onset of analgesia approximately 30 minutes. Lasts 3–4 hours.

Oramorph syrup	10 mg/5 ml, 100 mg/5 ml
Oramorph unit dose vial	10 mg/5 ml, 30 mg/5 ml, 100 mg/5 ml
Sevredol tablet	10 mg, 20 mg, 50 mg
Morphine suppository	10 mg, 15 mg, 20 mg, 30 mg

The latter is useful if the patient unable to swallow.

Usually started 4-hourly. After 48 hours the minimum total daily dose taken is divided by 2 and given as a sustained release formulation twice daily. The immediate release formulation is then used as required 4-hourly for breakthrough pain.

Once a steady state has been achieved this may remain static for weeks or months. If the cause of the pain is non-malignant this dosing regimen will suffice for a long period of time unless further physical damage takes place, e.g. further osteoporotic collapse of vertebral bodies. This may require specialist review by, for example, the orthopaedic service.

Sustained release

Onset of analgesia 1–2 hours. Lasts 12 hours.

MST Continus	5 mg, 10 mg, 15 mg, 30 mg, 60 mg, 100 mg, 200 mg
Oramorph SR	10 mg, 30 mg, 60 mg, 100 mg
MXL	30 mg, 60 mg, 120 mg, 150 mg, 200 mg
Morcap SR	20 mg, 50 mg, 100 mg

It is important to specify the precise formulation of morphine to avoid an immediate release drug being used in error 12-hourly or a slow release drug being used for breakthrough pain.

Diamorphine

This drug is only available in Britain and Canada. Its name is derived from its structure: There are two acetyl groups attached to a morphine molecule. See below for conversion from morphine dosing.

There is no advantage in giving this drug orally, but it is of great value if given by subcutaneous infusion. A high concentration may be dissolved into a small volume of Water for Injection or normal saline; therefore, a high dose can be infused into the sc layer. It is of particular value when the oral route cannot be used. Maximum concentration = 250 mg/ml. (see below for compatibility with anti-emetics).

Tramadol[2]

50–100 mg 4–6 hourly (o/im/iv)

Useful in SR formulation given twice daily. Arguably of limited use for long-term therapy, since it costs significantly more than the older drugs, but it may have a place in the transition period when analgesic requirements are increasing from weak to strong opioids. Caution must be exercised in patients prone to epilepsy.

Hydromorphone[3]

This has only recently been made available in Britain. It may be of value if there is a true morphine intolerance or allergy. As with morphine, the dose is titrated using the immediate release capsules. This can then be converted to the slow release formulation. It is seven times as potent as morphine; therefore, caution must be exercised when using in patients with no prior exposure to morphine because of the risk of respiratory depression.

Fentanyl TTS patch

This is another useful route of administration if the oral route cannot be used, and is better used once analgesic requirements have been established and are stable (see below).

Each patch releases a set amount of the drug per hour and each patch lasts for 3 days. For example a '25' patch will release 25 micrograms/hour of fentanyl. They exist as '25', '50', '75' and '100' patch. Occasionally there will be a need to use more than one patch. The disadvantage of the patch is that it is difficult to finely tune the analgesic requirements; it can take 12–18 hours for the plasma levels of the drug to peak and it can also take several hours for the plasma levels to drop in the situation of inadvertent overdosing.

Methadone[4]

This is a useful opioid to use if the patient is considered to have opioid-sensitive pain but appears to be morphine-resistant (sometimes called 'paradoxical pain'). Also it only needs to be given once a day.

The problem with this drug is that it takes much longer to be removed from the body (up to ten times longer than morphine). This means that higher doses are needed initially; then the dose needs to be reduced. It may take up to ten days to reach steady analgesic levels, and caution must be exercised to avoid respiratory depression.

Dosing plan

- Start with an initial dose that is one-tenth of the total daily morphine dose via the oral, subcutaneous or intravenous route.
- Allow the patient to have subsequent doses according to their level of pain. This should be no more frequent than every 3 hours. Typically the patient requires 3–8 doses for the first few days (3 doses, i.e. 8-hourly dosing is usual). The total daily dose may then be divided into a twice daily regime and make subsequent changes as one would with sustained release morphine.

Pethidine

This is not suitable for chronic use since it has a very short half-life of 2 hours and also it is metabolized by the liver to norpethidine, which can trigger epilepsy.

Conversion factors for morphine and diamorphine[5]

3 mg oral morphine ≈ 2 mg oral diamorphine ≈ 1 mg diamorphine by injection

> e.g. 15 mg oral morphine 4-hourly
> ≈ 10 mg oral diamorphine
> ≈ 5 mg diamorphine (im/sc) 4-hourly
> ≈ 30 mg diamorphine (sc infusion) over 24 hours

Compatibilty of diamorphine with anti-emetic agents

Compatible

Metoclopramide 5 mg/ml[6,7]
Methotrimeprazine 10 mg/ml[6]
Hyoscine hydrobromide 0.12 mg/ml[6,7]
Dexamethasone 1.6 mg/ml

Potentially incompatible

Haloperidol ≥ 2 mg/ml
Cyclizine ≥ 15 mg/ml
(Water for injection or 5% dextrose should be used to avoid precipitation)

Incompatible

Chlorpromazine

Prochlorperazine

Conversion dose from morphine to transdermal fentanyl

Morphine (mg/day)	Fentanyl patch
<135	'25'
135–224	'50'
225–314	'75'
315–404	'100'
405–494	'25' + '100'
...	...

Anti-emetic agents

Finally the pharmacology of anti-emetic agents will be discussed, since analgesics used or the pain itself may trigger nausea or vomiting which can sometimes distress the patient more than the pain itself, or may lead to dehydration and electrolyte imbalance.

Guidelines

Most anti-emetic drugs only have an effect for about 4 hours, yet their frequency of administration is limited to 3–4 times a day in order to minimize side-effects. Therefore if one agent appears inadequate it is worth considering alternating agents from different pharmacological groups. Also if a patient is feeling nauseated or is actively vomiting the oral route will be ineffective because the drug will not be absorbed. Causes of nausea and vomiting are illustrated diagrammatically in Figure 8.1 and appropriate anti-emetics are indicated.

Dexamethasone (steroid)

Up to 16 mg/day (o/im/iv)

Avoid after 2 p.m., when it may cause insomnia. Gradually reduce the dose to minimum effective dose. Stop after 7 days if no improvement on maximum dose.

Cyclizine (antihistamine)

50 mg   8-hourly (o/im/sc)

Domperidone (dopamine antagonist, prokinetic)

10–20 mg   8-hourly (o)

Less sedation or risk of extrapyramidal side-effects, such as oculogyric crisis, than other drugs in this class.

Metoclopramide (dopamine antagonist, prokinetic)

10–20 mg   8-hourly (o/im)

See under Domperidone for risks.

Prochlorperazine (dopamine antagonist)

5–10 mg   8-hourly (o)
3–6 mg   12-hourly (buccal)
12.5 mg   8-hourly (im)
25 mg   8-hourly (pr)

See under Domperidone for risks. Do not give subcutaneously (sc).

Methotrimeprazine (dopamine antagonist)

6.25–25 mg (o/sc)   8-hourly
25–100 mg/day   sedative dose

See under Domperidone for risks. Sedative therefore use at the lowest effective dose unless sedation required.

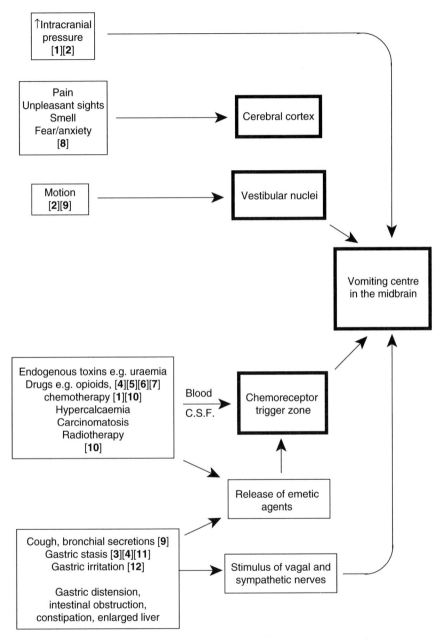

Figure 8.1 Causes and pharmacological control of nausea and vomiting. Key to anti-emetics: **1**, dexamethasone; **2**, cyclizine; **3**, domperidone; **4**, metoclopramide; **5**, prochlorperazine; **6**, methotrimeprazine; **7**, haloperidol; **8**, diazepam/midazolam; **9**, hyoscine; **10**, ondansetron; **11**, cisapride; **12**, antacids. (From *The Palliative Care Handbook*, 4th edn, 1998, courtesy of the Wessex Palliative Physicians)

Haloperidol (dopamine antagonist)

1.5–5 mg	nocté (o/sc)
2.5–5 mg/24 hours	via syringe driver (sc)

See under Domperidone for risks.

Diazepam (benzodiazepine)

2–15 mg total daily dose given up to 3 times a day.

Midazolam

10–30 mg/day	via syringe driver

Hyoscine (anticholinergic)

0.3–0.6 mg 6–8 hourly (sl/sc)	
0.8–2.4 mg/day	via syringe driver (sc)
0.5–1.5 mg/72 hours	by transdermal patch

Ondansetron (5HT3 antagonist)

8 mg	2–3 times daily (o/sc/im/iv)

Use prior to chemotherapy or radiotherapy.

Cisapride (5HT4 agonist)

10 mg	8-hourly (o)

Antacids

Proton pump inhibitor

Omeprazole 20 mg daily (o)

Prostaglandin analogue

Misoprostol 200 µg twice daily (o)

If caused by NSAIDs.

Summary
- The first goal of pharmacological control is to consider what aspect(s) of the pain is/are causing concern for the patient.
- One should select appropriate drugs, using their lowest effective doses to maximize their synergistic effects and minimize their side-effects.
- Side-effects are often significant enough to discourage the patient from continuing with the prescribed medication.
- Regular re-evaluation is required so that appropriate changes may be made quickly, giving the patient confidence in the efficacy of the treatment.

Acknowledgements

I would like to thank Wessex Palliative Physicians for permission to adapt their diagram on the causes of nausea and vomiting.

References

1. World Health Organization (1986) *Cancer Pain Relief.* Geneva: WHO.
2. Lee, C. R., McTavish, D. and Sorkin, E. M. (1993) Tramadol: a review. *Drugs*, 46, 313–40.
3. Steinberg, S. K. and Kornijenko, M. (1988) The role of hydromorphone hydrochloride. *Canadian Journal of Pharmacology*, 121, 182–6.
4. Sawe, J., Hansen, J., Ginman, C., Hartvig, P., Jakobson, P. A., Nilsson, M.-I., Rane, A. and Anggard, E. (1981) Patient-controlled dose regimen of methadone for chronic cancer pain. *British Medical Journal*, 282, 771–3.
5. Burne, R. and Hunt, A. (1987) Use of opiates in terminally ill children. *Palliative Medicine*, 1, 27–30.
6. Allwood, M. C. (1984) Diamorphine mixed with anti-emetic drugs in plastic syringes. *British Journal of Pharmaceutical Practice*, 6, 88–90.
7. Regnard, C., Pashely, S. and Westrope, F. (1986) Anti-emetic/diamorphine mixture compatibility in infusion pumps. *British Journal of Pharmaceutical Practice*, 8, 218–20.

9

Cognitive and behavioural pain management

M. Munafò

Introduction

The study of pain has, throughout its history, been beset with problems of definition. Pain itself has been variously described in physiological, somatic, cognitive, affective and cultural terms. The widely cited International Association for the Study of Pain definition of pain as 'An unpleasant sensory and emotional experience associated with actual or potential tissue damage, or described in terms of such damage', tacitly acknowledges the role personal meaning and subjective experience plays,[1] but at the same time the definition becomes largely meaningless by attempting to incorporate all possible facets of pain without sufficient analysis.

This problem of definition becomes apparent when the literature on pain is reviewed, as each author approaches his chosen problem with implicit assumptions about the nature of the phenomenon under study. When chronic pain is researched this problem is compounded – chronic pain is not simply the conjunction of pain and chronicity, although some would like to view it as such. The traditional conception of chronic pain as being definable simply by duration is misleading, as will be shown. Furthermore, the distinction between acute and chronic pain is not as clear as is often assumed. However, the dominant model of pain at present, gate control theory,[2] is essentially a model of acute pain, and it is by no means clear to what extent this model can be applied to a chronic setting.

The chronic pain syndrome

What is often examined in cases of chronic pain that present to a psychologist or behavioural scientist is, in fact, the chronic pain syndrome, a state of being characterized along certain behavioural, affective (emotional) and cognitive dimensions. Any physical/physiological dimension of pain is neither a necessary nor a sufficient condition for the existence of the syndrome. It is important to regard pain as a symptom rather than a disease; if anything is a disease it is the chronic pain syndrome, with chronic pain itself being a crucial symptom. It soon becomes clear that it is not possible to investigate simply the chronic pain feature of the syndrome, as several other factors are too intimately involved to be held constant. Typical features of the chronic pain syndrome include:

- reduced mobility
- reduced social activity
- depression
- aggressiveness
- negative thoughts about self
- negative thoughts about the future
- dependence on medication
- marital problems

To state the matter simply, the duration of chronic pain alone allows the development of maladaptive learning and changes in behaviour by means of psychological mechanisms. As has already been stated, part of the problem in the chronic pain syndrome is non-somatic in origin. It is generally the case that the pain begins acutely with some physical pathology; unfortunately, the point at which the patient can be described in terms of the chronic pain syndrome is not at all clear. In some cases the physical pathology remains but is intractable, whereas in others no physical pathology can be identified. In this discussion it will be assumed that all chronic pain patients who may benefit from cognitive and/or behavioural treatments display most or all of the features of the chronic pain syndrome to some degree.

Treatment

Treatment of the chronic pain patient has tended to proceed using isolated conceptions of the genesis of the chronic pain syndrome. Pharmacological and surgical treatments are widely used, but these have several drawbacks and assume some underlying physical pathology. It is still common for chronic pain patients who do not conform to this model to have their pain regarded as in some sense not real, despite overwhelming evidence to the contrary. At the risk of belabouring the point, it is essential that the chronic pain syndrome be regarded as not simply the result of some underlying physical pathology which remains unresolved. The placebo effect is now widely documented, and Bonica[3] estimates that one-third of chronic pain patients with mild or moderate pain respond positively to a placebo intervention. More active interventions have included attempts to manipulate levels of self-efficacy, several forms of relaxation, including biofeedback and hypnosis (discussed in another chapter), cognitive treatment to encourage positive coping strategies, and behavioural programmes based on an operant conditioning conception of the development of the chronic pain syndrome. All of these have met with success, and some encouraging results have been reported.

Information

For some time information-giving has been known to improve pain management, for example in the preparation for surgery to reduce postoperative pain and improve emotional well-being.[4] Information has also been shown to have an effect in experimental manipulations of pain.[5] This can be related to the self-efficacy theory of Bandura.[6] In acute pain, higher self-efficacy expectancies (i.e. the subject's own belief in his ability to manage his pain) are associated with better coping for experimentally induced pain. Self-efficacy is also predictive of management of acute clinical pain. In the case of the chronic pain syndrome, poor efficacy beliefs may be regarded as a cognitive barrier to normal function and pain management. Disability beliefs need to be reversed[7], and this is probably best done by facilitating performance accomplishments.[6] In other words, although verbal persuasion can be of use, the greatest increase in self-efficacy beliefs can be achieved by the subject performing some task which he previously believed himself to be unable to accomplish. Self-efficacy expectations have been shown to be predictive of both outcome in treatment and increase in exercise among chronic pain patients.[8,9] Therefore, if self-efficacy beliefs can be manipulated, improvement in function should become easier to achieve.

Cognitive management

Already several cognitive mechanisms have been identified as having some therapeutic value for chronic pain patients. Ciccone and Grzesiak[10] suggest that chronicity extends the opportunity for cognitive analysis, with irrational, negative beliefs being formed about the chronic pain and its implications. These authors argue that the cognitive style of chronic pain patients is characterized by:

- awfulizing — regarding events in the most negative possible light
- overgeneralizing — transferring the inability to do one task to other tasks
- low frustration tolerance — being highly irritated by minor setbacks
- external locus of control — the belief that events are beyond one's control

It is this shift in the cognitive style of the patient which is the cause of many of the emotional and physical problems associated with the chronic pain syndrome. It should be apparent that pain itself need only be an indirect cause of these problems. If we accept individuals as active participants in the nature of their experiences, then cognitive processes will have to play a central role in any understanding of chronic pain. The cultural, familial and personal meaning of the pain will have some effect on the cognitive style of the sufferer – to give an example, styles of pain complaint tend to be consistent within families,[11] so that it may be possible to speak of 'pain-prone' families. Global concepts, such as locus of control, learned helplessness and self-efficacy, although not identical, are in many ways related[6] and may be of central importance to any understanding of the chronic pain syndrome. Furthermore, the fine detail of the cognitive style of chronic pain patients may be necessary to explain many of the emotional and behavioural consequences of chronic pain.

Behavioural management

One treatment model for chronic pain patients which has produced some very positive results, and a certain degree of controversy, is that developed by Fordyce and his colleagues. This model maintains that the behaviours typical of the chronic pain patient lead to responses by others, and that these tend to be favourable. These favourable consequences of pain behaviours have been termed gain, and sub-divided into primary, secondary and tertiary gain.[12] The first refers to any intrapersonal, psychological mechanism for the reduction of unacceptable affect or conflict, the second to the interpersonal or environmental advantage supplied by the behaviour, and the last refers to any advantage that someone other than the patient may gain from the behaviour. The crucial notion here is that in some sense there may be an advantage to pain behaviour of the sufferer, such as avoidance of a disliked job. As a result the consequences of pain behaviour act as reinforcers, so that an operant conditioning model is appropriate to understanding how these behaviours (inactivity, pain complaint, dependency on medication, etc.) are produced, increased and maintained.[13] Operant conditioning is simply the extent to which behaviours change to fit their environment, so that any behaviour which provides an advantage (reinforcement, e.g. food) occurs increasingly often. In this way chickens learn to peck at buttons that release food.

It is important to realize that Fordyce is not suggesting that pain is produced by operant conditioning, but that pain problems are signalled by certain behaviours, and these behaviours, like all behaviours, are subject to specific influences, such as operant conditioning.[14] Table 9.1 shows the type of behaviours, typical of chronic pain patients, which may be susceptible to reinforcement.

Table 9.1 Common pain behaviours and potential reinforcers

Situation	Behaviour	Reinforcer/gain
Nociception	Reduce activity	Reduce nociception
Nociception	Pain medication	Reduce nociception/euphoria
Nociception	Limping/guarding	Sympathy/attention
Home environment	Pain complaint	Avoid stressors/housework
Work environment	Pain complaint	Avoid work
Doctor	Pain complaint	Medical attention
Lawyer	Pain complaint/inactivity	Financial reward
Spouse	Pain complaint/inactivity	Sympathy/attention

Behavioural treatment programmes based on these principles attempt to remove the connection between pain behaviour and reinforcement, instead encouraging reinforcement of well behaviours. This may operate on an inpatient or outpatient basis. For example:

Before treatment
Medication – received on demand or pain complaint.
Inactivity   – encouraged, e.g. 'lie down and rest your back'.
Activity   – discouraged, e.g. 'don't pick up that'.

During treatment
Medication – received at regular time intervals, NOT on demand.
Inactivity   – positively discouraged.
Activity   – encouraged, e.g. daily activity schedule, with
                 rewards.

It is crucially important to make sure that the patient understands the rationale behind this dramatic change in the treatment that they will be receiving. Also important is the role of the family, who must play a part in the treatment as it is they who, most likely, provide the reinforcement for the pain behaviours. Without the full cooperation of all concerned this approach is unlikely to meet with success.

Treatment programmes constructed around a behavioural theoretical framework have met with some success in reducing behaviours typical of the chronic pain syndrome, such as inactivity and excessive reliance on medication. The approach has been criticized on the grounds that it does not treat the actual pain but may only teach patients to be stoical. Fordyce and his colleagues[15] have responded by arguing that their principal objective is not to modify nociception but to render the patient functional by modifying the external expression of pain. Furthermore, there is substantial evidence for purely environmental reinforcers: if a supportive spouse is present the patient will rate his pain as higher, whereas with an unsupportive spouse the reverse is the case. In other words, the behaviour and complaint of the pain patient depends, to a degree, on whether the spouse is present and the nature of the patient–spouse interaction.[16,17] Exactly how effective cognitive and behavioural treatments are, however, remains unclear, and they are best used in combination with other treatments. Table 9.2 summarizes some recent research findings regarding the effectiveness of cognitive and behavioural therapy, although it is difficult to make comparisons across studies because of the different methodologies, interventions and patient groups included.

It is true that these programmes tend to be highly selective, and if they were not the success rate might be less, but there is still strong support for the efficacy of these treatment programmes and the theoretical foundation on which they are based. None the less, the actual pain of the patient is important and, indeed, this seems to be reduced as a result of these treatments, even though this is not a primary goal. It is also difficult to satisfactorily conclude that cognitive factors play no part: in the previous discussion of self-efficacy it was noted that performance accomplishments are most effective at altering self-efficacy beliefs, and

Table 9.2 Cognitive-behavioural management of chronic pain

Author	Year	Condition	No. patients	Treatment	Control	Assessment	Duration	Results	Analysis
Pilowsky et al.	1995	Chronic non-malignant pain	40	CBT + amitriptyline	Support + amitriptyline	Self-report pain and mood	8 weeks + 6 mth follow-up	No difference	n.s.
Richardson et al.	1994	Chronic non-malignant pain	109	CBT	None	Quality of life or return to work	12 weeks + 12 mth follow-up	Significant improvement	P<0.01
Newton-John et al.	1995	Chronic low back pain	44	CBT	Biofeedback + wait list group	Self-report pain and disab.	8 weeks + 6 mth follow-up	Significant improvement	P<0.01
Slater et al.	1997	Chronic low back pain	34	CBT	Medical care group	Self-report pain and mood	8 weeks + 6 mth follow-up	No difference, but improved	n.s.
Basler et al.	1997	Chronic low back pain	76	CBT + medical care	Medical care group	Self-report pain and disab.	12 weeks + 6 mth follow-up	Significant improvement	P<0.05
Vlaeyen et al.	1995	Chronic low back pain	71	Operant vs cognitive vs biofeedback	Wait list group	Observer rated behaviour	8 weeks + 12 mth follow-up	Significant improvement	P<0.01

much of the behavioural treatment depends on performance accomplishments. There is a need for research into the cognitive changes resulting from these programmes, although this is confounded by the fact that most programmes are not purely behavioural and rely to some extent on other psychological treatments. A different perspective may lead to unwarranted criticism, but may also illuminate important factors which had previously been ignored. Also, the primary goals of treatment will be different to the primary goals of research, so that there are certain ethical issues in research of this kind.

Research overview
Physiological correlates of psychological factors

So far this discussion has focused on the psychosocial aspects of the chronic pain syndrome. Lipman,[18] however, reports that peak B-endorphin concentration in cerebrospinal fluid is reduced in chronic pain patients. Further, this level increases when a placebo is administered to those patients that respond to placebo treatment. This indicates a biological basis for the analgesic placebo response in some chronic pain patients. The explanation proposed attempts to link these findings with gate control theory.[2] It seems that there will also be some psychological effects of placebo administration, and there are difficulties in attempting to separate psychological and physiological effects, which may act differentially depending on whether there is any organic pathology underlying the patient's pain.

Personality and emotion

Personality and mental illness has also been extensively researched in the chronic pain field. Benjamin[19] reports that 40% of psychiatric admissions have some kind of pain, with only half of these showing any relevant physical pathology. Chronic pain patients tend to show a range of organic and mental disorders which may or may not coincide. The most common mental illnesses exhibited by chronic pain patients are depressive or somatoform in origin, although in most studies there are problems of sample selection introducing biases, for example by using pain clinic patients. None the less, anxiety and depression are common features of the chronic pain syndrome, and in a sub-group of patients administration of antidepressants may resolve the pain.

Personality change is also thought to be common in chronic pain patients, and Deardorff[20] identified, through factor analysis of the Minnesota Multiphasic Personality Inventory, version 2 (MMPI-2), four factors related to chronic pain. These they labelled Psychological Dysfunction, Interpersonal Isolation, Psychomotor Retardation, and Physical Dysfunction. It is suggested in this study that these factors can be used to assess how far along the continuum towards chronic pain a patient has progressed. This notion of a continuum characterizing the chronic pain syndrome is useful, but there are problems here with the direction of causation. If we wish to talk of a 'pain-prone' personality these factors may have some causal influence on the development of chronic pain. Indeed, it may be possible to redescribe the factors so that they conform to the cognitive models already quoted. In this way, a patient may be at a higher risk of exhibiting specific symptoms of the chronic pain syndrome if they, for example, show low self-efficacy beliefs about resolution of their pain while they are in the sub-acute phase.

Problems of assessment

Unfortunately in the area of chronic pain there also tend to be some chronic methodological problems. Advances in assessment have not kept pace with advances in therapies and models of chronic pain. Pain is not the same as tissue damage, so that physical tests can only give a gross picture, but often a negative physical diagnosis leads to the clinician choosing a psychogenic diagnosis.[21] This simple dichotomy is hopelessly inadequate at encompassing the various causal factors in chronic pain. Measurements of pain behaviour alone could arguably be more objective, but there are few agreed examples of pain behaviour, and this approach would tend to neglect psychological factors. The conclusion must be that any adequate assessment of pain must be multidimensional in nature, and attempts have been made in this direction. For example, the McGill Pain Questionnaire[22] includes sensory, affective and cognitive questions. Unfortunately there is evidence that this still measures only one construct – a multidimensional questionnaire is not the same as a multiaxial one.[21] Advances in assessment are being made, but it is still dishearteningly common to find clinicians adhering to a strictly biomedical model, resorting to psychological models with a sense of failure.

There are also problems in the studies of the effectiveness of various interventions. If pain clinics are used to recruit subjects, these may not be representative of the entire chronic pain population. There is evidence for a higher incidence of depressive illness among pain clinic patients.[23] This selection bias is a particular problem in behavioural treatment models which have very stringent inclusion criteria. Comparison between studies is problematic if different criteria are used, and many patients who might provide interesting findings are lost because they do not meet the required criteria.[23] There is a need for some evaluation of patients who choose not to enter treatment and those who do not complete the course. For example, the goals of the clinic and the patient may be incompatible – behavioural clinics attempt to treat pain behaviours, while it is reasonable to expect most patients to hope for some treatment to alleviate their pain. These patients are lost to most studies.

Conclusion

So far this discussion has been an unashamed attempt to highlight the need for a broader understanding of the problem of chronic pain. This is not to say that there is no place for physiological findings. The dominant model of acute pain at present is gate control theory, and if this could be incorporated into the findings detailed already it would be most useful. Melzack and Wall[2,22] propose that the substantia gelatinosa acts as a gate to modulate patterns of activity before these influence the T cells. Patterns in the dorsal column activate brain processes that influence the properties of the gate, and T cells activate neural mechanisms which are responsible for response and perception. The central feature of this model is the gate, which may be opened or closed by both signals from afferent nerve fibres and descending messages from the cortex. If the gate is open the subject is more sensitive to pain, and vice versa. This model accounts for the moderate correlation between tissue damage and pain sensation.

Certain features of the gate control model, particularly the notion of descending messages influencing the gate, may allow an integration with psychological theories. The endorphin-mediated systems may be readily incorporated, and it is possible that the cognitive appraisal of the pain may influence the status of the gate. Since the model is primarily an acute one, it may be most useful in describing the initial stages in the development of chronic pain. The organic pathology results in significant levels of pain, and if self-efficacy beliefs are low this may serve to open the gate. Consequently the pain is maintained and the patient avoids activities which may serve to alleviate it. At this stage the behavioural model becomes appropriate, since the pain behaviours will result in some gain for the patient. As the chronic pain syndrome gradually develops the organic pathology becomes less important and psychosocial and behavioural factors begin to dominate. Therefore at this stage it is more appropriate to treat these factors. If any organic pathology does remain there may be the added benefit of these treatments acting to close the gate, and thereby directly influencing the physiological substrate of the pain.

What is evident is that chronic pain is now capable of being treated very effectively, with many previously untreatable patients now leading almost normal lives as a result of interventions based on psychological models. That these treatments proceed using a variety of models should not be seen as a criticism, but there are good grounds for believing that many of the results can be conceptualized using a common cognitive framework. Furthermore, it may be possible to integrate this framework with physiological models such as gate control theory. If the transition from acute to chronic pain is seen as a continuum, the primary influences may vary in importance along this continuum. This allows for pre-emptive intervention to prevent the development of chronic pain, and the possibility of the 'pain-prone' individual being characterized by certain cognitive styles allows for a prediction of those at risk of suffering from chronic pain.

Many of the suggestions given here are based on speculation, and there is a need for research into the effects of specific cognitions and cognitive styles, particularly in treatments that do not specifically target these. There is also the question of how, if at all, these cognitions may influence the physiology of pain, and this is likely to be the most difficult question. The finding that higher self-efficacy benefits in experimentally reduced pain are partly reversible by naloxone[8] gives a certain amount of hope that this question may be answerable. It should be realized that it may in fact be possible to explain the same phenomenon at different levels, perhaps cognitive and physiological, without necessarily having to choose between these. What is of paramount importance, however, is that a broader conception of the problems and issues involved here is adopted. Part of the reason chronic pain patients feel isolated and anxious is that in our society there exist no cultural resources for coping with chronic pain.[24] The only understanding of pain is based on the belief that it is something which will go away, and if this is not the case patients need to know that this is not necessarily abnormal.

Summary

- Psychological does not mean 'not real'; psychological variables will have physiological correlates which may explain the mechanism of these effects.
- Pain is multidimensional, and includes emotional, cognitive and behavioural aspects, as well as physiological ones.
- Treatments may focus on one or several of these aspects; for example, cognitive treatments attempt to modify negative beliefs about the pain, the self, the future, etc.
- Behaviours are influenced by expectations and the consequences of these behaviours, as well as by the environment.
- Effective pain management will have to operate at several levels, concurrently tackling nociception, pain behaviours, pain cognitions, mood, and so on.

References

1. Wall, P. D. (1983) Pain as a need state. *Journal of Psychosomatic Research*, 27(5), 413.
2. Melzack, R. and Wall, P. D. (1965) Pain mechanisms: a new theory. *Science*, 150, 971–9.
3. Bonica, J. J. (1979) re: The relation of injury to pain (Letter). *Pain*, 7, 203–7.
4. Egbert, L. D., Battit, G.E., Welch, C.E. and Bartlett, M. K (1964) Reduction of postoperative pain by encouragement and instruction of patients: a study of doctor–patient rapport. *New England Journal of Medicine*, 270, 825–7.
5. Staub, E. and Kellet, D. S. (1972) Increasing pain tolerance by information about aversive stimuli. *Journal of Personality and Social Psychology*, 21, 198.
6. Bandura, A. (1977) Self-efficacy: toward a unifying theory of behavioural change. *Psychological Review*, 84, 191–215.
7. Elton, D., Stuart, G. V. and Burrows, G. D. (1978) Self-esteem and chronic pain. *Journal of Psychosomatic Research*, 22, 25–30.
8. Lackner, J. M., Carosella, A. M. and Feuerstein, M. (1996) Pain expectancies, pain, and functional self-efficacy expectancies as determinants of disability in patients with chronic low back disorders. *Journal of Consulting and Clinical Psychology*, 64(1), 212–20.
9. Jensen, M. P., Turner, J. A. and Romano, J. M. (1991) Self-efficacy and outcome expectancies: relationship to chronic pain coping strategies and adjustment. *Pain*, 44, 263–9.
10. Ciccone, D. S. and Grzesiak, R. C. (1984) Cognitive dimensions of pain. *Social Science and Medicine*, 19(12), 1339–45.

11. Craig, K. D. (1984) Psychology of pain. *Postgraduate Medical Journal*, 60, 835–40.

12. Bokan, J. A., Ries, R. K. and Katon, W. J. (1981) Tertiary gain and chronic pain. *Pain*, 10, 331–5.

13. Fordyce, W. E., Fowler, R. S., Lehmann, J. F. and DeLateur, B. J. (1968) Some implications of learning in problems of chronic pain. *Journal of Chronic Disorders*, 21, 179–90.

14. Fordyce, W. E. (1984) Behavioural science and chronic pain. *Postgraduate Medical Journal*, 60, 865–8.

15. Fordyce, W. E., Roberts, A. H. and Sternbach, R. A. (1985) The behavioural management of chronic pain: a response to critics. *Pain*, 22, 113–25.

16. Romano, J. M., Turner, J. A., Jensen, M. P., Friedman, L. S., Bulcroft, R. A., Hops, H. and Wright, S. F. (1995) Chronic pain patient–spouse behavioral interactions predict patient disability. *Pain*, 63, 353–60.

17. Paulsen, J. S. and Altmaier, E. M. (1995) The effects of perceived versus enacted social support on the discriminative cue function of spouses for pain behaviors. *Pain*, 60, 103–10.

18. Lipman, J. J., Miller, B. E., Mays, K. S., Miller, M. N. *et al.* (1990) Peak B endorphin concentration in cerebrospinal fluid: reduced in chronic pain patients and increased during the placebo response. *Psychopharmacology*, 102(1), 112–16.

19. Benjamin, S., Barnes, D., Berger, S., Clarke, I. *et al.* (1988) The relationship of chronic pain, mental illness and organic disorders. *Pain*, 32, 185–95.

20. Deardorff, W. W., Chino, A. F. and Scott, D. W. (1993) Characteristics of chronic pain patients: factor analysis of the MMPI-2. *Pain*, 54, 153–8.

21. Turk, D. C. and Rudy, T. E. (1987) Towards a comprehensive assessment of chronic pain patients: a multiaxial approach. *Behaviour Research and Therapy*, 25, 237.

22. Melzack, R. and Wall, P. D. (1982) *The Challenge of Pain*. Harmondsworth: Penguin.

23. Turk, D. C. and Rudy, T. E. (1990) Neglect factors in chronic pain treatment outcome studies – referral pattern, failure to enter treatment and attrition. *Pain*, 43, 7–25.

24. Hilbert, R. A. (1984) The acultural dimensions of chronic pain: flawed reality construction and the problem of meaning. *Social Problems*, 31(4), 365–78.

Alternative treatments: transcutaneous electrical nerve stimulation (TENS)

J. Trim

Transcutaneous electrical nerve stimulation (TENS) can be applied to a vast variety of pain conditions, both chronic and acute in origin. TENS has been used in the outpatient setting by physiotherapists and chronic pain relief units for many years and the number of patients receiving TENS appears to be increasing. This has an impact on the nurses working in the acute setting, as more patients come into hospital using TENS or TENS is applied while the patient remains in hospital.

This chapter will explore some of the conditions in which a nurse working in the acute setting may see TENS as part of a patient's pain management programme, giving the nurse a greater understanding of why TENS has been chosen as a form of pain relief and assisting the nurse in the management of patients using TENS.

The chapter will discuss the action of TENS, the relevant indications and contraindications, and the conditions in which TENS has been found to be of benefit. The equipment used will be explored and, finally, the information that the user will require to achieve maximum benefit will be discussed. A patient information sheet is also included.

The intention is to offer the reader an aid to understanding the basic principles of TENS; the chapter does not equip the reader with the knowledge to prescribe or apply TENS to patients.

Introduction

Transcutaneous electrical nerve stimulation (TENS) is a safe, effective form of drug-free pain relief, involving passing an electrical current across the skin via electrodes. It has been suggested that the gate control theory of pain[1] can explain its effect, by serving to close the gate, and thereby preventing the pain messages from reaching the brain. Its effect may also be explained in part by the endogenous opioid system, with TENS increasing the patient's level of endorphin activity, therefore providing pain relief. The sensation felt by the patient from TENS is usually described as tingling or vibrating; it should not be unpleasant or painful, as this will reinforce the pain messages.

The origins of TENS can be traced back to the ancient Egyptians and Romans, who used electric fish to stimulate the skin and relieve pain.[2] The development of TENS to relieve pain came about after the publication of Melzack and Wall's gate control theory in 1965,[1] which suggested a role for the central summation of peripheral nerve messages. Since then TENS has been used to relieve pain in both chronic and acute pain problems.

The equipment

TENS units are small, portable and battery operated, consisting of three main parts – a stimulator box (the energy source), lead wires and electrodes (see Figure 10.1).

Stimulator box

The stimulator box will normally have the following controls:

- On/Off switch and intensity control.
- Frequency control (pulse rate).
- Width control (pulse duration).
- Mode selector.
- On multi-channel units an intensity control is provided for each channel.

Pulse frequency is measured in Hertz (Hz) and is the number of stimulation cycles delivered per second. The low frequency range is from 1 to 50 Hz, while 50–100 Hz is considered high frequency. The lowest effective frequency should be used. Frequencies above 100 Hz have not been found to increase the effectiveness of TENS.

High frequency stimulation is aimed at activation of myelinated cutaneous sensory fibres. Low frequency stimulation is aimed at activation of muscle afferent or muscle cells, thereby evoking muscle afferent inputs to the central nervous system (CNS). Low frequency stimulation also has an acupuncture-like action.[3]

Current intensity is measured in milliamperes (mA) and is the strength of the electric stimulation applied to the electrodes. Current intensity for TENS usually ranges from 10 to 60 mA.

Pulse duration is measured in milliseconds (ms), and is the length of time each pulse cycle lasts. TENS duration is set between 0.05 and 0.5 ms.[2]

Lead wires and electrodes

A pair of insulated wires connect the stimulator and the electrodes. Two or more electrodes may be used depending on the type of TENS unit and the pain problem.

There are two types of electrode normally available, carbon rubber pads and self adhesive disposable pads, and these come in a variety of shapes and sizes. Carbon rubber pads are applied to the skin using conductive gel and fixation tape. The use of saline gel is essential in order to achieve good electrical contact between the electrode pad and the skin. The gel must be evenly applied over the whole surface of the pad. Only gel designed for use with TENS should be used. Other types of jelly such as ECG jelly are not recommended as they may contain a higher concentration of sodium chloride, which can cause irritation to the skin. The pads are secured in place by adhesive tape or pre-shaped adhesive pads designed to fit over the electrode pad. Self-adhesive pads are stored on waxed paper when not in use, and these can be purchased directly from TENS companies.

Electrodes, conductive gel or tape must be changed if there is any sign of skin irritation.

Cost and acquisition

TENS units are commercially available and the price for a basic unit will be approximately £35. Some companies are willing to loan TENS units to patients for a trial period. TENS machines are also advertised in the media, and patients can purchase the unit directly from the company.

Indications for TENS

There is evidence to suggest that TENS works best when patients have had careful explanation prior to commencement of use,[4] and continuing support during the first few months will ensure that the patient achieves maximum benefit.

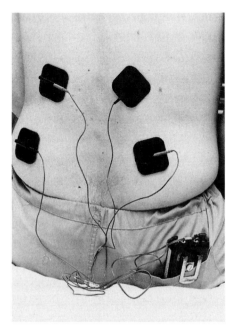

Figure 10.1 TENS equipment in use

Success rates vary, with between 30% of chronic pain and 70% of acute pain problems reporting good pain relief with TENS. It is difficult to accurately predict which patients and what types of pain respond well to TENS.

There appears to be conflicting information as to whether TENS is or is not effective, and many of the studies conducted contradict each other, not only as to the percentage of successful pain relief per pain condition, but also the types of condition for which TENS is most effective.

However, as TENS appears to be effective when the pain is localized, and as TENS is a safe, non-invasive method of pain relief, it is often worth a trial period.

Examples of conditions in which TENS may be of benefit include:

- Chronic or acute back pain.
- Sciatic pain.
- Arthritis.
- Neck pain, e.g. whiplash.
- Fractured ribs.
- Phantom limb pain.
- Trigeminal neuralgia.
- Headache due to tension, fever or hangover.
- Migraine and cluster headache.
- Dysmenorrhoea.
- Childbirth.
- Angina.
- Muscle spasm.
- Surgical and traumatic injury acute pain associated with surgery and traumatic injuries.
- Peripheral neurogenic pain, in conjunction with medication.[5]

Note that TENS should not be used as the sole treatment for moderate to severe pain (e.g. in the case of surgical acute pain).

TENS should not be used in the following circumstances:

- If a cardiac pacemaker has been fitted.
- Before the 37th week of pregnancy, except on medical advice.
- Over a metal prosthesis.
- If allergic to conductive gel or electrodes.
- On skin lesions, rashes or open wounds, or over carotid sinuses or the throat.
- In the bath or shower.
- While operating hazardous machinery or driving.

Patients must be cooperative and able to understand the application of TENS, as this will increase the effectiveness of TENS. The physiotherapist or nurse who has been trained to apply TENS must explain the TENS unit to the patient and how and when to apply the electrodes.

In recent years some hospitals have developed special TENS fitting clinics within the chronic pain relief unit. These units tend to be run by nurses specially trained in the application of TENS. Teaching and education enable the patient to manage the TENS on a daily basis and increase the success rate of TENS.

Before TENS is used, the light-touch sensation over the area to be stimulated should be examined, as there must be functioning, normal light-touch receptors and fibres in the area being stimulated in order for TENS to be effective.

Where light-touch sensation is disturbed, the electrodes should be applied as close to the disturbed area as practical. The pulse width and pulse rate should be adjusted until the stimulation is felt to be uncomfortable, after which the intensity should be decreased until it becomes entirely pleasant.[6]

There should be no burning or pricking elements to the sensation and, if there is, first the pulse width and then the pulse intensity control should be turned down until the sensation is pleasant and is felt continuously.

Placement of electrodes

There needs to be a period of trial and error when placing the electrode pads at the commencement of treatment, to find the optimal placement site. This needs to be clearly explained to the patient in order to ensure that TENS is given an opportunity to work.

There are four main anatomical sites where TENS electrodes can be placed. These are: the painful area, the peripheral nerve, the spinal nerve root and specific points, such as acupuncture, trigger and motor points. Irrespective of the site chosen, stimulation will ultimately result in the passage of afferent information into the central nervous system.[7] Painful area placement is the most commonly used technique. There are a number of placement leaflets available from TENS companies to assist with the placement of the electrode pads.

There is evidence to suggest that TENS should be used for no more than one hour at a time, with a minimum 30 minute rest period between applications when used for chronic pain problems.[7] This reduces the possibility of skin irritation or muscle fatigue if using acupuncture-like TENS.

There are acute pain conditions which warrant continual use of the TENS unit, as the TENS will only be required for a relatively short time. There are a number of studies that suggest that TENS should be considered as a supplement to routine postoperative pain management[7] in conditions such as cholecystectomy, spinal fusion or thoracotomy, and in the management of labour pain.

The electrode pads are placed approximately 1.5 cm either side of the incision when used for postoperative pain relief.[8]

The overall package of TENS treatment may influence the patient's self-report of pain and treatment outcome, regardless of the actual effectiveness of TENS. Opinion as to this effectiveness is divided: There are some studies which suggest that TENS is no better than placebo TENS. One series of systematic reviews concludes that TENS does not provide pain relief for postoperative pain, labour pain and, possibly, chronic pain,[9] while another concluded that TENS was effective in a variety of acute pain conditions and back pain.[10] Conflicting reviews highlight the difficulty when assessing the effectiveness of TENS as a treatment for pain. Many health care professionals suggest that TENS is beneficial for patients, whether treating a physiological or psychological component of pain, and as such should not be dismissed without consideration.

TENS can be applied to a variety of pain conditions, both acute and chronic in nature, although it would appear that lack of knowledge regarding its use is the main barrier to utilization of this form of pain relief.

Assessment of the patient's suitability, and a trial period of TENS, is essential to maximize the likelihood of a positive outcome.[4] This, combined with educational programmes for health care professionals who care for patients using TENS, is vital to the success of this method of pain relief.

Patient information

The following is an example of a patient information sheet that should be given to the patient to keep for future reference.

What is TENS?
- *TENS stands for Transcutaneous Electrical Nerve Stimulation. It is a safe, effective form of drug-free pain relief, involving passing an electrical current across the skin via rubber or disposable electrodes. It works by preventing pain messages reaching the brain and, therefore, can provide pain relief.*

Is TENS a cure for pain?
- *No. Using TENS helps treat the symptom of pain, but it does not treat the cause; in other words, it may help ease the pain, but it won't cure the cause of your pain. The cause of your pain should be diagnosed before using TENS.*

Will TENS work for me?
- *It is not possible to predict who will do well with TENS, as every person is different. Unfortunately, it is a question of 'try it and see'. You may find it provides a lot of relief, or it may not help you much.*

What are the benefits of TENS?
- *It may help you cut down on your painkillers.*
- *It may help you lead a more active life with less pain.*
- *You can control when, where and how much you use it.*
- *TENS has no adverse side-effects if it is used as you have been advised.*

What does it feel like?
- *Using TENS should be comfortable. It will feel like a mild background tingling or buzzing, and not at all unpleasant.*

How do I use it?
- *You will be shown by the nurse how to use the machine and where the electrodes should be sited to provide maximum benefit.*

How long do I use the machine for?
- *This will vary from person to person, but it is likely that the machine will need to be used for up to 6 hours a day.*

- *Some people find greatest benefit using TENS in a single session, while others prefer using it intermittently throughout the day.*
- *Lifestyle factors will determine the use of TENS; for example, it may help to use TENS prior to increased activity, maintaining its use while remaining active.*

When should TENS not be used?
- *Do not use in the bath or shower.*
- *Do not wear in bed.*
- *Do not use before the 37th week of pregnancy, except on medical advice.*
- *Do not place the electrodes on broken skin or over the throat or carotid sinus.*
- *Do not use if you have a cardiac pacemaker.*
- *Do not place the electrodes over a metal prosthesis.*
- *Do not use when operating hazardous machinery or driving.*

Using TENS
- *Plug the ends of the wires into the self-adhesive electrode pads.*
- *Plug the wire into the machine with the machine turned off.*
- *Attach the electrodes to your skin in the position shown to you.*
- *Switch the machine on and adjust the settings to suit your personal daily needs.*
- *Switch the machine off before removing the electrodes.*

Care of the machine after use
- *Prolong the life of the self-adhesive pads by storing them in the refrigerator overnight. If they lose some stickiness, wipe the surface of the pads with a damp cloth before applying them to the skin.*
- *Rubber pads need to be washed in soapy water when removed, and allowed to dry before reapplying.*
- *Wipe the wires gently with a clean damp cloth regularly to prevent the build-up of dust.*
- *Store the machine in the case provided when not in use.*
- *It is important to pay special attention to the area the pads are applied to. The area should be washed in warm water and dried well before application of the pads, and after they are removed.*
- *In some cases, people can develop sensitivity to the pads. If this does occur, it may be possible to use a different manufacturer's product that may have different constituents to the rubber.*

Summary
- TENS can be used to manage pain problems, both acute or chronic in nature, in a wide variety of settings.
- Opinion as to the effectiveness of TENS is divided.
- Patients should be aware that TENS will not be of benefit to every patient in every situation. Initial assessment of patient suitability and trial of TENS increases the likelihood of a positive outcome.
- There are contraindications for TENS, such as skin sensitivity or damage, the presence of metal prostheses or cardiac pacemakers, etc.
- Education programmes for health care professionals are important to the success of TENS.

References

1. Melzack, R. and Wall, P. D. (1965) Pain mechanisms: a new theory. *Science*, 150, 971–9.
2. Salerno, E. and Willens, S. (1996) *Pain Management Handbook*. London: Mosby.
3. Melzack, R. and Wall, P. D. (1994) *Textbook of Pain*. Edinburgh: Churchill Livingstone.
4. Mitchell, A. and Kafai, S. (1997) Patient education in TENS pain management. *Professional Nurse*, 12, 804–807.
5. Bushnell, M., Marchaud, S., Tremblay, N. and Duncan, C. (1991) Electrical stimulation of peripheral and central pathways for the relief of musculosketal pain. *Canadian Journal of Physiology and Pharmacology*, 69, 697–703.
6. Diamond, A. W. and Coniam, S. W. (1996) *The Management of Chronic Pain*, 2nd edn. Oxford: Oxford University Press.
7. Walsh, D. (1997) *TENS Clinical Applications and Related Theory*. Edinburgh: Churchill Livingstone.
8. McCaffrey, M. and Beebe, A. (1994) *Pain: Clinical Manual for Nursing Practice* (UK edition). London: Mosby.
9. Carroll, D., Moore, A., Tramer, M. and McQuay, H. (1997) TENS in labour pain: a systematic review. *British Journal of Obstetric Gynaecology*, 104, 169–75.
10. Reeve, J., Menon, D. and Corabian, P. (1996) TENS: a technology assessment. *International Journal of Technology Assessment and Health Care*, 12, 299–324.

11
Alternative treatments: acupuncture

G. T. Lewith

Introduction

Acupuncture (or needle puncture) is a European term invented by Willem Ten Rhyne, a Dutch physician who visited Nagasaki in Japan in the early part of the seventeenth century. The Chinese describe acupuncture by the character 'Chen', which literally means 'to prick with a needle'.

Acupuncture has a recorded history of about 2000 years, although some authorities claim that it has been practised in China for much longer. The Chinese believe that stone knives or sharp-edged tools were used some 4000 years ago to puncture and drain abscesses; these instruments were called 'Bian' stones. The character 'Bian' means the use of a sharp-edged stone to treat disease. The modern Chinese character 'Bi' describes a disease of pain and is almost certainly derived from the use of 'Bian' stones for the treatment of painful complaints.

The origin of Chinese medicine is complex, and acupuncture represents only one facet of the development of the traditional Chinese medical system. The first recorded attempt at conceptualizing and treating disease dates back to about 1500 BC; tortoise shells with inscriptions were thought to have been used for divination and also in the art of healing. The philosophical basis for much of very early Chinese medicine seems to have been to seek harmony between the living and their dead ancestors, and the good and evil spirits that inhabited the earth.

The first known acupuncture text is the *Nei Ching Su Wen*. This book is also known by a variety of alternative titles such as the Yellow Emperor's Classic of Internal Medicine, or the Canon of Medicine. The initial section of the *Nei Ching Su Wen* involves a discussion between the Yellow Emperor, Huang Ti, and his Minister Ch'I Pai, which lays down the philosophical framework of traditional Chinese medical thought. The authorship of the *Nei Ching Su Wen* is attributed to Huang Ti, but there is some doubt as to whether he actually existed and a great deal more uncertainty as to who wrote the book. It was probably written by a variety of people and seems to date from the Warring States period (475–221 BC).

The Western doctor observes the facts before him and uses the current physiological theories to explain them. Chinese medicine is based on a much wider worldview, but one that is more difficult to justify and almost impossible to test within the context of an empirical experiment. These ideas are woven into a complete system based on a philosophy different from that of Western medicine. In essence, the ideal of health is perfect harmony between the forces of Yin and Yang. However, this state is rarely attained and most of us exist in a state of fluctuating health: one day we feel well and the next day less well. All of us are in a state of change, but it is only when this change causes persistent and irreversible disharmony that it results in established disease.

Acupuncture needles and moxibustion

As acupuncture developed, the Bian stones were discarded and needles of stone and pottery were developed. Eventually metal needles appeared, and these took the form of the classical 'nine needles', each with a different function – a sort of Chinese physician's surgical kit. The main needle now used for acupuncture is the filliform.

A discussion of the development of acupuncture is incomplete without mentioning moxibustion. This is the burning on or near the skin of the herb moxa. The Chinese character 'Chiu' is used to describe the art of moxibustion, and literally means 'to scar with a burning object'. Moxibustion does not now involve scarring, but moxa is still used to provide local heat over acupuncture points and is made from the dried leaves of *Artemisia vulgaris*.

The evolution of acupuncture points and channels

Acupuncture points are undoubtedly the end product of millions of detailed observations and, as they were developed, so each of them was given a Chinese name, which implied its functional and clinical importance. Common painful diseases consistently cause painful points to emerge in well-defined anatomical locations. When such a point is stimulated, the pain can be alleviated, hence the idea of a point for treating pain. From this simple beginning it is easy to see how a system of acupuncture points evolved for the management of painful conditions.

Acupuncture points were subsequently grouped into a system of channels which run over the body; the channels are said to conduct the flow of vital energy through the body. Furthermore, each channel, or group of acupuncture points, was designated with the name of an organ and said to represent the functional integrity of that organ (for example, see Figure 11.1). The Chinese believed that if an organ were malfunctioning, then this would lead to an abnormal flow of vital energy in the channel representing that organ. The therapeutic implication of these assumptions is that the judicious selection of acupuncture points on the appropriate channels could then be used to normalize the flow of vital energy within them and subsequently return the organ to normal function.

The development of acupuncture

Over the ensuing centuries, acupuncture and moxibustion became part of a sophisticated medical system. Medical colleges were established in China during the sixth century AD, and many well-illustrated and refined texts were published about these therapeutic techniques. During the Ming Dynasty (AD 1368–1644) the first consistent contacts were established with Europe. With the traders went priests to convert the 'heathen', and it was through these priests, and the various physicians who visited China, that the idea of acupuncture began to filter through to the West. The Jesuits were particularly active in collating and disseminating information, but the process was far from one-sided, as the Jesuits also introduced Western science to China. Dominique Parrenin, a missionary, translated a textbook of anatomy into Mandarin, but the

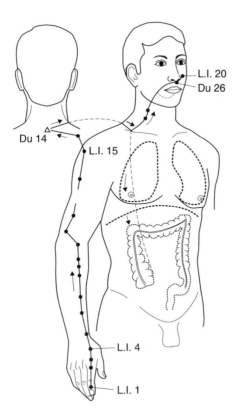

Figure 11.1 The large intestine channel. (Derived from Bowsher, 1998[2])

Emperor banned this from general circulation as he recognized that many of the Western concepts contradicted those of traditional Chinese medicine.

The Ching Dynasty (AD 1644–1911) was a time of chaos for the Chinese. The Ching Emperors regarded acupuncture as a bar to progress and, in 1822, a government decree eliminated acupuncture from the curriculum of the Imperial Medical College. In spite of its decline, acupuncture remained the medicine of the masses. The Imperial denigration of acupuncture reflected not only the poor standard of practice, but also the fact that some of the educated Chinese were looking to the West for progress.

Western medical colleges were set up by the missionaries, the first being in Canton. The missionaries translated Western medical books into Chinese and in 1886 began to print the *China Medical Missionary Journal*, which was the first scientific journal in China. Another medical college was established shortly afterwards in Tientsin and there was a gradual increase in the number of Western-trained Chinese doctors. Finally, in 1929, the practice of acupuncture was outlawed in China.

The Communists actively cultivated Chinese enthusiasm for various forms of traditional medicine such as acupuncture. They realized that there were few or no medical services in the 'liberated areas' during the Revolution, and that the traditional methods were cheap and acceptable to the Chinese peasants. Consequently, acupuncture gained new momentum and, during the early 1950s, many hospitals opened up clinics to provide, teach and investigate the traditional methods of medicine, the main research institutes being in Peking, Shanghai and Nanking. This renaissance of acupuncture, combined with a sophisticated scientific approach, has allowed the development of many new methods in this therapy and has undoubtedly provided one of the many stimuli for current Western enthusiasm.

Acupuncture in the West

It is probable that acupuncture has been known and used in the West since the seventeenth century, but its first recorded use was by Dr Berlioz, at the Paris Medical School in 1810, who continued to use acupuncture, and claimed great success with it. Acupuncture is not new to England, the first known British acupuncturist being John Churchill who, in 1821, published a series of results on the treatment of tympany and rheumatism with acupuncture. In 1823 acupuncture was mentioned in the first issue of *The Lancet* and, in 1824, Dr Elliotson, a physician at St Thomas's Hospital, London, began to use this method of treatment. In 1827 he published a paper describing the treatment of 42 cases of rheumatism by acupuncture, and concluded that this was an effective therapeutic method for such problems.

Within the context of Western medicine, the development of acupuncture points on the body demonstrates an interesting story of rediscovery. Over the past 50 years many Western physicians have discovered, independently, that pressing, stimulating or injecting various superficial body points can help to relieve pain, particularly musculo-skeletal pain. These points are not necessarily at the site of pain, but are often at distant areas. For instance, cervical spondylosis frequently presents with pain over the shoulder or scapular region. On close examination, it is frequently possible to define the origin of the pain and demonstrate that the neck is the cause of the problem. However, injection or stimulation of the painful points around the scapula will often relieve the pain and free neck movement. Melzack[1] correlated these trigger points with acupuncture points, and found that most trigger points were already well known and described as acupuncture points. There have been a number of attempts to understand the existence of trigger points, but as yet there is no clear explanation of this phenomenon. It is interesting to note that the Chinese realized this fact some 3000 years ago, and the *Ling Shu* summarizes this approach when it says: 'In pain puncture the tender point'.

Traditional Chinese medicine

While accepting that many doctors practise needle puncture simply by selecting and needling the local tender points which relate to painful areas, it would be inappropriate and historically incorrect to ignore the origins of this system of medicine. Therefore it is important to examine the conceptual and diagnostic systems used within Traditional Chinese Medicine (TCM) in order to provide the basis for a more complete understanding of this therapy.

Western medicine presupposes that a human being is Cartesian in nature: the body represents one functioning system, and the mind another. It accepts that each system is interrelated, but essentially it sees disease as either physical or mental. The Chinese assume that the body is whole, and that each part of it is intimately connected, with each organ having a mental as well as a physical function. In a diagnostic and conceptual sense, TCM is holistic as it assesses the patient as a complete functional unit.

The Chinese system of medicine suggests that health is achieved and disease prevented by maintaining the body in a balanced state; this concept could be applied both to individuals and to society as a whole. In individual terms, ancient Chinese physicians preached moderation in all things, such as food and alcohol, and also suggested that normal activities should include mental as well as physical tasks. The wealthier Chinese visited their doctors when they were well, paying a retainer to the doctor as long as they remained healthy; if they became ill, the doctor lost his fee.

The cornerstone of health, within the context of TCM, is a normal fluctuating balance of Yin and Yang. If such balance ceases to exist, then the Chinese believe that external agents (or pathogens) could invade the body and cause disease. The essential principle of TCM is to specify the exact nature of the imbalance between Yin and Yang, and the pathogen causing the trouble. Acupuncture points can then be selected to correct these pathological processes and, as the natural forces of the body become balanced, the disease will be eliminated. The art of TCM is to particularize this imbalance accurately so that it can be corrected. The patient is then treated by using specific acupuncture points on the body or ear in order to re-balance the body. In general terms, the patient will give a better response if very few acupuncture points are used; therefore, if the acupuncturist can select the appropriate points with accuracy, the patient is likely to show a swift and effective response to treatment. In acupuncture, and indeed within all the complementary therapies, the opposite applies. The patient's failure to respond or improve may well suggest that too much therapy has been given.

The diagnostic and therapeutic principles of Yin and Yang and the pathogens are based on a system of anatomy and physiology peculiar to TCM. The anatomy of TCM is represented by the acupuncture points and the channels that connect them. Its physiology has many similarities to that of Western medicine; most of the organ functions defined in the *Nei Ching Su Wen* correlate well with modern physiology.

The heart is said to dominate the circulation of blood. The *Nei Ching* says: 'The heart fills the pulse with blood … and the force of the pulse flows into the arteries and the force of the arteries ascends into the lungs'. This seems to be a clear description of the double circulation of blood; the idea of blood circulated in this way was peculiar to Chinese medicine until it was 'rediscovered' by William Harvey in the early seventeenth century.

In TCM the major bodily functions are built around the five main organs – the heart, the lungs, the kidneys, the liver and the spleen. In Western medicine these organs are of vital importance, but not to the same extent as in TCM. The Chinese call them the five 'Zang' (or solid) organs and it is the system of the five 'Zang' organs that controls the body's health. Each of the 'Zang' (solid) organs is linked to a 'Fu' (hollow) organ. For instance, the kidney is linked both structurally and functionally to the urinary bladder. In Eastern and Western medicine both organs are accepted as controlling the production and passage of urine; the channels representing the kidney and urinary bladder are also paired as vital energy is said to flow from one channel to the other. TCM assumes that the emotions are governed by individual organs; it does not consider the brain and subconscious as discrete entities. Therefore, the body and mind are a real part of the same functional system. Each organ is given a particular emotion; for instance, the liver is said to be the organ affected by anger or irritability.

The Chinese believed that the force behind biological functions occurring in any living tissue necessitated vital energy, or 'Qi', which has both substantive and functional elements. The substantive or material form of 'Qi' is represented by normal body nutrients such as food or gaseous exchange. The non-substantive form is the real but elusive concept of a vital force, and goes some way to explaining why an otherwise healthy individual feels full of energy one day and drained and rather unproductive the next.

Disease results when the body is weakened and unable to resist the onslaught of pathogens. In Chinese medicine the agents that cause disease are given the names of meteorological conditions: an infection (often associated with a fever) is called a disease of heat, and a chronically painful joint is usually a disease of cold. These pathogens allow diseases to be grouped according to their broad symptoms.

Other factors may also cause disease, such as worry or eating contaminated food. The *Nei Ching* states that excessive grief, anxiety and over-thinking will cause a tumour (cancer). In fact, this is mirrored by an observation made by the Roman physician, Galen, that those with a 'melancholy' disposition are predisposed to cancer, and this idea has been supported by some recent studies which suggest that if a woman has a breast removed for cancer, she will survive longer if she is of a happy and relaxed disposition. The traditional Chinese ideas about pathogens, both internal and external, would seem to have some degree of validity when analysed in an objective manner with the aid of modern scientific and epidemiological techniques.

One of the most difficult skills for the practitioner of traditional Chinese medicine is to define the specific organ affected by any particular disease. As with all systems of medicine, a detailed history often gives a very clear indication as to the diagnosis. If the acupuncturist understands the functions ascribed to each organ by the Chinese, then this will provide an essential and irreplaceable starting point from which a diagnosis can be made.

As well as observing and palpating the diseased area of the body, the ancient Chinese also palpated the pulse and looked in detail at the tongue. Pulse palpation was achieved by feeling the radial pulse at three positions on each wrist, and by noting the pulse characteristics at the superficial and deep sites at each of these. The superficial pulse can be palpated at approximately systolic pressure and the deep pulse at approximately diastolic pressure. There are therefore six pulses at each wrist, three superficial and three deep. There are 12 main organs in the Chinese medical system, and each of these is represented by one of the pulses at one of the wrist positions. It is unclear how the system of pulse diagnosis came into existence, but it had been refined and classified in detail by 500 BC. This method of diagnosis allows the whole body to be assessed and it also defines the relative balance between each of the organs. In addition, pulse diagnosis is said to give a clear idea of the type of disease process and pathogen causing that disease in any individual patient.

Acupuncture treatment

The diagnosis of a particular problem does not tell the acupuncturist where to place a needle; a set of therapeutic rules must be applied to solve that problem. To a large degree all medical systems are based on clinical experience, and acupuncture is no exception to this general rule. The rules of point selection may be based on a wide range of approaches to acupuncture. The simplest, and most obvious, is the use of acupuncture in acute or chronic pain. In this instance, points may be selected purely by localizing the most tender trigger zones and needling the tender points alone.

However, in many diseases, and in the case of pain, associated symptomatology may be present. This might include anxiety and/or depression, or irritable bowel and indigestion, which can sometimes be produced by analgesic or non-steroidal anti-inflammatory agents. In such instances it may be difficult, if not impossible, to select points purely based on the patient's localization of pain. In disease processes, such as asthma, point selection cannot be based on tender point localization and does require some knowledge of TCM and the empirical rules of point selection.

Many complementary medical techniques are considered safe simply because they are natural. When inserting needles into the body, care must be taken and there are some well recorded adverse reactions that do occur as a consequence of acupuncture. Probably the most common is fainting, but if needles are improperly sterilized then cross-infection with both bacteria and viruses (hepatitis/HIV) have been recorded. Modern disposable needles, however, mean that this should not happen in properly regulated practice. The puncturing of vital organs is also a potential adverse reaction to acupuncture, and a number of cases of pneumothorax have been recorded. The information we have suggests that acupuncture is indeed far safer than many conventional treatments, but caution and proper training is needed as adverse reactions do occur.

Acupuncture treatment, particularly for pain, almost invariably involves more than one treatment. It is usual to consider that a course of acupuncture will be given, comprising six to eight treatments, and that improvement will be progressive. If the pain is the result of chronic degenerative pathology, then it is likely that acupuncture treatment will need to be repeated periodically, every 3, 6 or 12 months, if the patient is to obtain a good and prolonged clinical result. Sometimes, very severe pain simply does not respond, while occasionally problems that should respond to very simple acupuncture just do not seem to.

The physiological mechanism of acupuncture

Much has been written about the physiological mechanisms of acupuncture in pain, and I would refer the reader to two reviews should they wish to learn more about the neurophysiology of acupuncture.[2,3] There is a large amount of evidence which looks at how acupuncture may affect the nervous system. While initially the gate control theory was thought to explain the basis of acupuncture analgesia, the picture soon broadened to include work on the natural opioid system. It is now clear that there are both neurological and neurohumoral mechanisms through which acupuncture is mediated. However, most of this information has been obtained from animal studies involving acute pain. It is still questionable how much of this data relates to chronic human pain, which is the situation in which acupuncture is most frequently used.

Acupuncture points

Acupuncture works through acupuncture points and is said to be only effective if these are needled correctly. Many of these points correlate closely with small nerve bundles that penetrate the fascial lining of muscles, or are very close to the nerve bundles that surround major blood vessels. The sympathetic nervous system is almost certainly involved in acupuncture, and we can also demonstrate that acupuncture points are areas in which the electrical skin resistance is far lower than the surrounding normal skin. Information about the meridians, and how they might be explained neurologically, is less clear. There is some evidence suggesting that the acupuncture meridians may have an autonomic connection, while other theories point to their correlation with the lymphatic system.

Figures 11.2, 11.3 and 11.4 are drawn from Bowsher's excellent chapter on the mechanism of acupuncture,[2] and explain in some detail how the neurological and neurohumoral mechanisms combine, initially at a

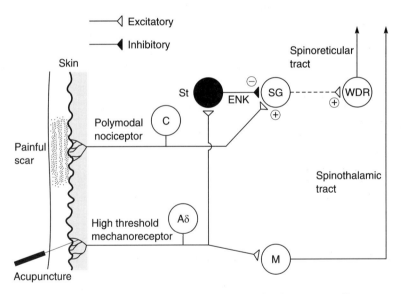

Figure 11.2 Mechanism of segmental acupuncture. The C primary afferent polymodal nociceptor projects to substantia gelatinosa (SG) cells in the superficial dorsal horn; these generate further impulses that pass to, or perhaps disinhibit, wide dynamic range (WDR) (or convergent) cells whose axons pass up to the brain in the spinoreticular tract where they are eventually interpreted as painful.

The Aδ primary afferent pinprick receptors project both to marginal cells (M), which project up to the brain in the spinothalamic tract carrying information about pinprick that will become conscious, and to enkephalinergic stalked cells (St), which can release enkephalins (ENK) that inhibit SG cells, thus preventing information generated by noxious stimulation being transmitted further. (Derived from Bowsher, 1998[2])

segmental level (Figure 11.2) and then through both the serotonergic (Figure 11.3) and adrenergic (Figure 11.4) systems. It is abundantly clear that while acupuncture starts off as a peripheral and potentially painful stimulus, its first effects are neurological, stimulating small, myelinated afferents in the skin and muscle. Segmental acupuncture clearly works

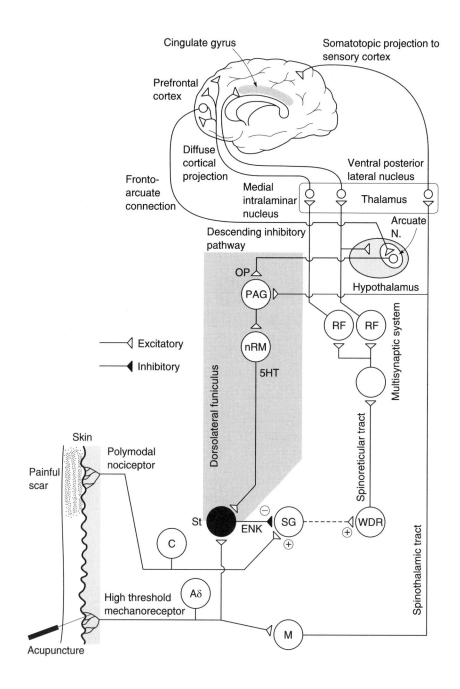

through an inhibitory enkephalin-based system, whereas acupuncture in a segment that is different to that in which the pain lies has an effect through far more general neurohumoral mechanisms involving the release of beta-endorphin, met-enkephalin and two descending neurological mechanisms (one of which is serotonergic and the second of which is adrenergic).

Acupuncture in pain

Lewith and Machin[4] were the first to review the randomized clinical trials on acupuncture. They suggested a model for evaluating the clinical effects of acupuncture in which a placebo effect would occur in 30% of patients, a real treatment effect in 70% of patients and the use of sham acupuncture or random needling (that is, the insertion of acupuncture needles into non-acupuncture points inappropriate for the condition being treated) would have an effect in approximately 50% of patients entered into any study. The evidence from controlled trials was conflicting and confusing, largely because the majority of them were so poor, statistically, that it was impossible to draw any reasonable conclusions from the published data in the early 1980s. Three more recent systematic reviews of the use of acupuncture in pain have subsequently been published. Ter Riet[5] analysed 51 controlled clinical trials looking at the effectiveness of acupuncture in pain according to a list of predefined methodological criteria. The results from the better constructed studies were very contradictory, and the authors concluded that the efficacy of acupuncture in chronic pain was limited. Patel[6] looked at 14 trials and came to an entirely different conclusion, suggesting that most of the results in their systematic review favoured acupuncture. A more recent systematic review of acupuncture studies in back pain by Ernst[7] also supports Patel's view, in that he suggests that acupuncture is effective in neck pain.

The main problem that occurs in amalgamating the results from different acupuncture studies is the very many different types and

---

Figure 11.3 Serotonergic mechanism of acupuncture. Pinprick information is carried up from marginal cells (M) to the ventroposterior lateral thalamic nucleus, whence it is projected to the cortex and becomes conscious; but in the midbrain these axons give off a collateral branch to the periaqueductal grey matter (PAG). The PAG projects down to the nucleus raphe magnus (NRM) in the midline of the medulla oblongata, and this in turn sends serotonergic (5HT) fibres to the stalked cells (St). The latter inhibit substantia gelatinosa cells (SG) by an enkephalinergic mechanism (ENK), and so prevent noxious information arriving in C primary afferent nociceptors from being transmitted to wide dynamic range (WDR) cells deep in the spinal grey matter, which send their axons up to the brain (reticular formation, RF). OP = opioid peptides. The PAG is also influenced by opioid endorphinergic fibres descending from the arcuate nucleus in the hypothalamus, and the hypothalamus in turn receives projections from the prefrontal cortex. (Derived from Bowsher, 1998[2])

techniques of acupuncture that are used clinically. Studies on back pain may, for instance, include some groups of patients who have received minimal acupuncture (a needle inserted into the skin a millimetre or two) while other groups of patients may have received electrical stimulation

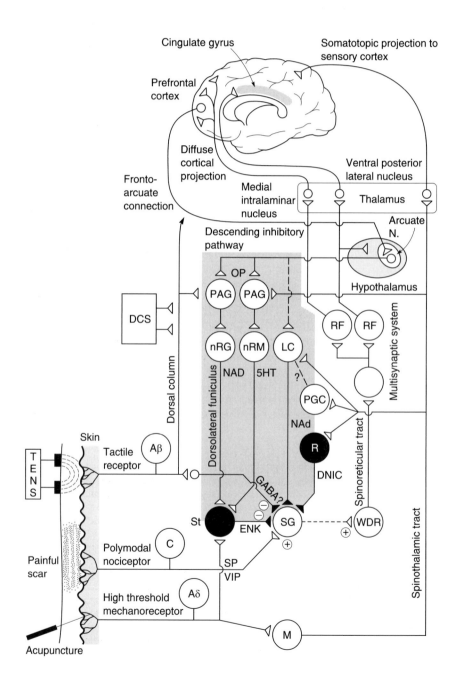

for half an hour associated with deep needling. As yet we do not have enough information to decide which is the 'best' acupuncture treatment in any particular condition and so the whole idea of amalgamating different acupuncture studies into systematic reviews is worrying.

Acupuncture itself is a treatment that has been used widely for over 3000 years; the treatment itself has 'stood the test of time' and must now be exposed to proper controlled trials. For the purposes of answering the question 'How effective is acupuncture' it is, therefore, reasonable to rely largely on the conventional model of the randomized controlled trial for an answer. This, in spite of the disadvantages and problems associated with randomized controlled trials in acupuncture, provides us with some interesting reading.

Table 11.1 documents the use of acupuncture in headache; only a small number of studies have been done, usually involving very few patients. Most of the studies are non-significant and suggest that acupuncture is of limited value.

Table 11.2 analyses the effect of acupuncture in facial pain. In the majority of studies, acupuncture appears to be better than the comparable placebo or control treatment (where one is used). Again, however, only very few of the studies have appropriate statistical methodology applied to them so that it is difficult to answer questions about its effectiveness conclusively.

Table 11.3 documents studies of acupuncture in neck pain, while more have been reviewed by Ernst.[7]

Some of the studies noted in Table 11.4 were used by Ernst et al. in their meta-analysis of back pain, and these generally show that acupuncture is more effective than the placebo or control with which it was compared.

Similarly, the studies reported in Table 11.5, which refer to musculoskeletal pain, show a general improvement, compared to the placebo or control group in pain report and, in some cases, mobility.

Figure 11.4 Adrenergic mechanism of acupuncture. Marginal cells (M), activated by Aδ pinprick receptors, in addition to their projections to the ventral posterior lateral nucleus and the PAG, also send axon branches to the following. (a) Subnucleus reticularis dorsalis (R) in the caudal medulla oblongata. Descending projections from this structure bring about inhibition of noxiously generated information arriving at the spinal cord (SG) in C nociceptors. This is the diffuse noxious inhibitory control mechanism. (b) Nucleus paragigantocellularis lateralis (PGC), which indirectly brings about noradrenergically mediated inhibition at spinal cord level. (c) The locus coeruleus at the junction of medulla oblongata and pons. Its noradrenergic axons (NAD) are directly inhibitory to those spinal neurones with which they enter into synaptic contact. OP = opioid peptides, DCS = dorsal column stimulation.
The figure also includes the Aδ primary afferent tactile receptor, which projects to the dorsal column and in addition, via an interneurone, to the SG cells. Thus activation of the tactile receptor sends impulses to the dorsal column and also, via the interneurone, leads to an inhibition of the SG cells, probably through the release of α-aminobutyric acid (GABA). The latter action will prevent information generated by noxious stimulation being transmitted further. (Derived from Bowsher, 1998[2])

Table 11.1. Trials of acupuncture in headache

Author(s)	Year	Condition treated	Type of trial	No. of pts	Type of acu.	Length/no. of treatments	Control group	Assessment	Duration	Results	Analysis
Borglum Jensen et al.	1979	Unspecified headache	Crossover	29	MS 1 needle	1 × 20 min	Skin touched by needle	Frequency of attacks, analgesia intake	2 mth	↓frequency of headaches in both groups. Acu. ↓ analgesia intake	N/S
Loh et al.	1984	Migraine	Crossover	48	MS. Local and distal points	2 min, variable no.	Medical treatment	Frequency, severity, duration of attacks	3 mth	Imp. in 60%	N/A
Dowson et al.	1985	Migraine	RC SB	48	CA body and seg. points	6 × 10 min	Mock TENS	Pain diary, analgesia intake	2 yr	Acu. 20% more effective	N/S
Vincent	1989b	Migraine	RC SB	30	CA MS Local and distal points	15 min 6 × weekly	Sham acu.	Severity, frequency of attacks, analgesic intake	6 wk 4 mth 1 yr	Pain reduction both groups	
Hesse et al.	1994	Migraine	RC DB	85	TP needling	6–8 × weekly	Point touched with blunt end of needle	Pain diary, severity and frequency of attacks	17 wk	Significant↓ frequency in both groups No difference between groups	$P<0.01$ N/S
Johansson et al.	1976	Tension	SB	33	CA MS	Not stated	Sham acu.	Not specified	8 wk	Acu. had a better effect than sham acu.	N/S
Borglum Jensen et al.	1977	Myogenic	U/C	21	MS 1 point	1 × 20 min	None	EMG recordings	1 day 1 mth 4 mth	60% imp. EMG showed decrease in postural activity	N/S

Author	Year	Condition	Design	N	Type	Treatment	Control	Outcome measures	Follow-up	Results	Significance
Ahonen et al.	1983	Myogenic, tension	U/C	22	CA	10 min × 4	Physio, U/S	Pain, VAS, EMG recording	2 mth	Similar pain relief and alteration EMG in all groups	N/S
Hansen and Hansen	1985	Tension	RC Crossover	18	CA MS	6 needles 2 × weekly for 3 weeks	Sham acu.	Pain scores, pain index	15 wk	Significant reduction pain scores	$P<0.05$
Vincent	1990	Tension	Single case/time series	14	CA	MS 15 min 8 × weekly	Sham acu.	Pain scores, pain diaries	8 wk 4 mth	>50% reduction in pain scores both groups	N/S
Carlsson and Sjölund	1994	Tension and neck pain	U/C	62	CA	7–8 times weekly	Physio	Pain intensity, muscle tenderness	17 wk	Reduction in both groups	N/S
Tavola et al.	1992	Tension	RC	30	CA	8 × 20 min	Sham acu.	Frequency, severity, duration, headache index, analgesia intake	1 mth 6 mth 12 mth	Both groups ↓frequency and analgesia intake	N/S

acu., acupuncture; CA, classical acupuncture; DB, double blind; imp., improvement; MS, manual stimulation; N/A, not applicable; N/S, not significant; RC, randomized controlled; SB, single blind; seg., segmental; U/C, uncontrolled; U/S, ultra sound; VAS, visual analogue scale.
Source: Based on Hester, J. (1998) In: Filshie, J. and White, A. (eds) Medical Acupuncture: a Western Scientific Approach. Edinburgh: Churchill Livingstone.

Table 11.2. Trials of acupuncture in facial pain

Author(s)	Year	Condition treated	Type of trial	No. of pts	Type of acu.	Length/no. of treatments	Control group	Assessment	Duration	Results	Analysis
Raustia et al.	1985	TMJ dysfunction	RC	50	Seg. and distal	20 min × 3	Standard stomato-gnathic treatment	Clinical dysfunction index	1 wk and 3 mth	Both groups imp. at 1 mth	N/S
Raustia and Pohjola	1986	TMJ dysfunction	RC SB	50	Seg. and distal	20 min × 3	Standard stomato-gnathic treatment	Painful movement of mandible	1 wk and 3 mth	Dental treatment better initially, no difference at 3 mth	N/S
List and Helkimo	1987	Chronic facial pain, mandibular dysfunction	U/C	10	MS EA	10 min × 8	None	Clinical index dysfunction, VAS, analgesia intake	3 mth and 7 mth	Subjective imp. in all	N/A
Johansson et al.	1991	Facial muscular pain	R	45	Local and distal	30 min × 6	Occlusal splint or untreated	Pain score, dysfunction score	3 mth	Both treatments reduced subjective dysfunction score	N/S
List and Heikimo	1992	Cranio-mandibular disorders	R	80	Local and distal	30 min × 6	Occlusal splint or untreated	ADL/VAS, pain diary, examination	1 yr	Both groups significant benefit; no difference between treatment groups	N/S

ADL, Activities of Daily Living; EA, electroacupuncture; R, randomized; other abbreviations as Table 11.1.
Source: Hester (1998)[8].

Table 11.3. Trials of acupuncture in neck pain

Author(s)	Year	Condition treated	Type of trial	No. of pts	Type of acu.	Length/no. of treatments	Control group	Assessment	Duration	Results	Analysis
Coan et al.	1982	Neck pain	R	37 30	CA	3/wk < 10	No treatment	Pain score, analgesia intake, activity levels	12 wk	80% imp. 40% ↓ pain score 54% ↓ analgesia intake, 32% increase activity	N/A
Loy	1983	Cervical spondylosis	R	60	EA	30 min 3 × weekly for 3–6 wk	Physiother.	Pain score neck movement	6 wk	EA 87% imp. Physio 54% imp. EA produced earlier imp.	N/A
Petrie and Langley	1983	Chronic cervical pain	R pilot	13	CA	20 min MS 2 × weekly for 4 wk	Mock TENS	PRS	1 mth	Acupuncture better than placebo	P < 0.01
Petrie and Hazelman	1986	Chronic cervical pain	RC	26	CA	20 min MS 2 × weekly for 4 wk	Mock TENS	VAS, MPQ, analgesia pain diary, neck movement	1 mth	No significant imp. in acu. group. Trends in daily activity and pill count	N/S
Peng et al.	1987	Neck and shoulder pain	U/C	37	EA tender points	20 min<15 2 × weekly	U/C	Hypnotic profile	Not stated	50% long term imp.	N/A
Lundeberg et al.	1988	Chronic head and neck pain	U/C	177	Local and intraseg. points	2/weekly × 10	Superficial acupuncture	Pain scores	2 yr	Pain score reduced by acupuncture in 56%	N/A
Thomas et al.	1991	Chronic cervical OA	R crossover	44	CA MS	1 × 40 min	Sham acu. diazepam, placebo	VAS, intensity and unpleasant-ness	3 wk	Significant ↓ pain and unpleasantness in acu. group	P<0.05 compared with placebo

EA, electroacupuncture; MPQ, McGill Pain Questionaire; OA, osteoarthritis; PRS, pain rating scale; other abbreviations as Table 11.1.
Source: Hester, 1998⁸.

Table 11.4. Trials of acupuncture in back pain

Author(s)	Year	Condition treated	Type of trial	No. of pts	Type of acu.	Length/no. of treatments	Control group	Assessment	Duration	Results	Analysis
Edelist *et al.*	1976	Low back pain	R SB	30	EA	3 × 30 min	Sham acu.	Pain relief, range of movement, neurological testing	1–3 wk	40% improvement in sham group, 46% in acu. group	N/S
Fox and Melzack	1976	Low back pain	R crossover	12	MS	3 min 3 × weekly	TENS	MPQ	4 mth	Pain relief >33% in 75% acu. group 66% TENS group	N/S
McDonald *et al.*	1983	Low back pain	R SB	17	Superficial acu., EA	4–6 × 20 min	Mock TENS	VAS, activity ratings, mood, pain relief	6 wk 6 mth	Significant benefit of acu. in pain relief, activity, and overall severity	P<0.01
Mendelson *et al.*	1983	Chronic back pain	DB crossover	95	CA, MS	1 × 30 min	Intradermal injection 2% lignocaine into non-acu. points	Pain score	3 mth	↓ pain score 26% acu. group, 22% control group	N/S
Lehmann *et al.*	1986	Low back pain	R	54	EA	2 × weekly for 3 wk	TENS, mock TENS	VAS, disability rating, physical measures	3 wk	No difference between 3 groups, trend towards less pain with acu.	N/S

Author	Year	Condition	Design	N	Intervention	Duration	Control	Outcome measure	Follow-up	Results	Significance
Garvey et al.	1989	Low back pain	R DB	63	MS, TP	1 treatment	Lignocaine inj, lignocaine with steroid, vapo spray and acupressure	VAS	2 wk	All groups improved	N/S
Thomas and Lundeberg	1994	Low back pain	R DB	40	MS EA 2 Hz EA 80 Hz	1 × 30 min	No treatment	Activity level, mobility, verbal pain rating	6 wk 6 mth	At 6 wk all groups significantly improved at 6 mth EA 2 Hz group only	N/S

Abbreviations as Tables 11.1, 11.3.
Source: Hester, 1998[5].

Table 11.5. Trials of acupuncture in musculoskeletal pain

Author(s)	Year	Condition treated	Type of trial	No. of pts	Type of acu.	Length/no. of treatments	Control group	Assessment	Duration	Results	Analysis
Gaw et al.	1975	Chronic OA pain	R DB	40	CA	8 × 30 min	Sham acu.	Joint tenderness, VRS, mobility, range of movement	3 wk	Significant imp. pain and mobility in both groups	N/S
Moore and Berk	1976	Chronic shoulder pain	R SB	42	CA	1 × weekly	Needle strapped to skin	Pain score, range of movement	3 wk	Significant imp. in pain in both groups	N/S
Godfrey and Morgan	1978	Musculo-skeletal pain	R DB	193	CA	3–5 treatments	Sham acu.	Pain score	3 wk	↓ pain in 63% of acu. group, 54% sham group	N/S
Berry et al.	1980	Shulder cuff lesions	R DB	60	CA	5 × weekly	Steroid inj., physio., NSAID, placebo pill	VAS, movement, comparative assessment	4 wk	All groups improved, no difference between them	N/S
Lundeberg	1984	Myalgia	R crossover	36	EA	2 × weekly for 3 wk	TENS, vibratory stimulation, placebo pill	VAS	3 wk	> 50% pain relief in 40 % of treated patients, 20% placebo group	N/A
Emery and Lythgoe	1986	Ankylosing spondylitis	DB crossover	10	EA	3 × 20 min	Sham acu.	Pain score and stiffness	9 wk	No significant effect on pain, stiffness improved in both groups	N/S

Author	Year	Condition	Design	N	Type	Treatment	Control	Outcome measures	Duration	Results	Significance
Christensen et al.	1992	OA knee	R SB crossover	29	MS	20 min 2 × weekly for 3 wk, then monthly	No treatment	Range of movement, pain score, analgesia intake	40 wk	↓ pain score, analgesia intake and ↑ movement	$P<0.03$
Deluze et al.	1992	Fibromyalgia	R SB	70	EA	6 × 2 weekly	Sham acu.	Pain threshold, analgesia intake, VAS, pain score, sleep quality, morning stiffness	3 wk	Significant difference for 5 out of 8 outcome measures	$P<0.03$
Molsberger and Hille	1994	Chronic tennis elbow	R SB	48	Non-seg. distal points	5 min × 1	Needle placed on skin	Pain relief	72 h	75% reported 50% pain relief	$P<0.01$
Takeda and Wessell	1994	OA knee	R SB	40	MS	3 × weekly for 3 wk	Sham acu.	PRS, OA index, pain threshold	3 wk	Reduction of pain, stiffness and physical difficulty in both groups	N/S

VRS, Verbal Rating Scale; NSAID, non-steroidal anti-inflammatory drug; other abbreviations as Tables 11.1, 11.3.
Source: Hester, 1998*.

It is interesting to note that acupuncture is now considered to be part of physiotherapy, and is used primarily as a physiotherapy technique for pain relief. The clinical evidence relating to acupuncture, particularly when one looks rigorously at the controlled trials is, to say the least, flimsy. Nevertheless, acupuncture is widely used in NHS pain and physiotherapy clinics in spite of the apparent lack of evidence.

Conclusion

Acupuncture is a fascinating therapeutic intervention, with its well-defined roots in traditional Chinese medicine. The technique has been known in the West for the past 300 years and is now widely used as a method of pain relief. While we have a clear understanding of how it may be acting neurophysiologically, the clinical data to support its use in chronic pain is not as powerful as it might be. Further more detailed research is desperately needed.

Summary
- Acupuncture involves the insertion of needles into strategic body and ear points (acupuncture points).
- Traditional Chinese Medicine is a philosophical and conceptual model that underpins our understanding of health and disease. It is used as the diagnostic and therapeutic basis for acupuncture and other Chinese remedies such as the prescription of Chinese herbal preparations.
- Channels of meridians link acupuncture points in an 'energetic sense' and allow the insertion of needles to have an effect on the body and organs within the traditional Chinese model of illness.
- Acupuncture is used in the West largely to treat pain, but it can also be used to treat a variety of 'internal diseases' such as asthma and nausea.
- Traditional Chinese diagnosis involves specifying the person's vital energy (Qi) through their history, pulse and tongue. This then forms the diagnostic basis that an acupuncturist will use and the subsequent point prescriptions they use for therapy.
- Acupuncture treatment works in stages and usually a course of 8–10 treatments is required. It lasts for a variable period of time (usually months).
- Acupuncture research has defined clear mechanisms through which acupuncture will affect the neurological and neurohumeral pathways that are involved in chronic and acute pain.
- Clinical research indicates that acupuncture is probably effective in pain, but further studies are required in this complex field which represents a challenge for clinical research.

References

1. Melzack, R., Stillwell, D. and Fox, E. (1977) Trigger points and acupuncture points for pain: correlations and implications. *Pain*, 3(3), 3–23.

2. Bowsher, D. (1998) The mechanisms of acupuncture. In: Filshie, J. and White, A. (eds), *Medical Acupuncture, a Western Scientific Approach*. Edinburgh: Churchill Livingstone.

3. Lewith, G. T. and Kenyon, J. (1984) The physiological and psychological explanations for the mechanism of acupuncture as a treatment for chronic pain. *Social Science and Medicine*, 19, 1367–78.

4. Lewith, G.T. and Machin, D. (1983) On the evaluation of the clinical effects of acupuncture. *Pain*, 16, 111–27.

5. Ter Riet, G., Kleijnen, J. and Knipschild, P. (1990) Acupuncture and chronic pain: a criteria-based meta-analysis. *Journal of Clinical Epidemiology*, 43, 1191–9.

6. Patel, M., Gutzwiller, F., Paccaud, F. and Marazzi, A. (1989) A meta-analysis of acupuncture for chronic pain. *International Journal of Epidemiology*,18, 900–6.

7. Ernst, E. and White, A.R. (1998) Acupuncture for back pain: a meta-analysis of randomized controlled trials. *Archives of Internal Medicine* , 158, 2235–41.

8. Hester, J. (1988) Acupuncture in clinical research methodology. In: Filshie, J. and White, A. (eds), *Medical Acupuncture, a Western Scientific Approach*. Edinburgh: Churchill Livingstone, pp. 319–40.

12

Alternative treatments: relaxation and hypnosis

M. Munafò

The use of relaxation therapy has become increasingly popular in recent years, while hypnotherapy, although also gaining in popularity, often suffers from a number of misconceptions about its nature and function. This chapter aims to outline the benefits that may be obtained by the use of relaxation and hypnosis in chronic pain, and suggested mechanisms which may underlie their efficacy. Those interested in a more detailed description of the various techniques available should refer to *Psychological Approaches to Pain Management*.[1]

Relaxation

There are three mechanisms that may be influenced by relaxation methods, all of which may be regarded as potentially relevant in the case of chronic pain. These are:

- sympathetic autonomic nervous system arousal
- muscle tension
- central nervous system/cortical activity

Sympathetic arousal

When faced with threat, our bodies react by increasing activation in the sympathetic nervous system, as well as with a release of hormones from the pituitary and adrenal glands, increasing blood pressure and breathing rate, diverting blood flow to the striated muscles, increasing adrenaline secretion, and so on. This 'fight or flight' response prepares the organism for physical exertion and is, therefore, a perfectly appropriate reaction to physical threat. Unfortunately, our bodies are unable to distinguish physical threat from emotional or psychological threat (i.e. stress), so that exactly the same reaction occurs when we are anxious, for example, about a forthcoming examination, when the response is much less likely to be appropriate.

Chronic pain is an example of a condition that frequently provokes anxiety, distress and so on. In these cases we would expect a sympathetic nervous system reaction, similar to that described above. If this persists over time the stress-related illnesses which may, in part, be caused by this reaction may develop, with attendant physical and psychological outcomes.

Muscle tension

All striated muscles must maintain a certain level of activity, or tension, in order to maintain tone (and thereby posture). However, it is possible for excessive activity to result in excessive tension, which is felt subjectively, unlike background tension, which passes unnoticed. This may be the result of anxiety or psychological stress, or may be caused by incorrect posture, guarding and so on.

Both of these types of cause are common in the case of chronic pain, where excessive muscle tension may often be a secondary cause of pain in itself.

Cortical activity

Background neural activity in the brain can be measured, crudely, by means of an electroencephalogram (EEG), using electrodes placed on the scalp. This provides a rough picture of the level of activity in the brain, in real time, and specific patterns of such activity have been identified and associated with subjective, psychological states. The pattern of cortical activity for a sleeping person, for example, is quite different to that of a waking person, while a relaxed person will show a different pattern of activity to an anxious, active person.

Generally speaking, increased cortical arousal (i.e. an EEG output with a higher frequency of spikes) is associated with intense emotion, in particular negative intense emotion. This, in turn, makes it difficult for the individual to relax or sleep, since high levels of EEG activity are incompatible with sleep, which may further exacerbate the anxiety or distress subjectively felt.

Methods of relaxation

The majority of methods of relaxation act by reducing the level of sympathetic nervous system activity or the degree of muscle tension, although there is evidence that cortical activity may also be modified directly by certain forms of relaxation (as opposed to indirectly, as a result of relaxation modifying other factors, which in turn modify cortical arousal).

Muscle relaxation is designed to reduce the degree of muscle tension in the subject, and may be either active or passive. In active muscle relaxation, groups of muscles are systematically tensed and then relaxed, with the participant focusing on the sensations that occur before, during and after each round of tension and release. The muscle group is tensed for a few seconds (5–6) and then relaxed for about four times as long (20–25 seconds). This provides an immediate benefit but also, more importantly, teaches the participant to distinguish between excessive muscle tension and relaxation. The process may be repeated for each muscle group and, after all muscle groups have been tensed and relaxed in this way, the participant will be in a relaxed state, commonly evincing reduced levels of pain in the case of chronic pain patients.

Passive muscle relaxation has a similar goal to active muscle tension, but omits the active tensing of muscle groups, instead relying on the individual facilitating the relaxation to play a more active, verbal role. Again, emphasis is on increasing the participant's subjective awareness of the different sensations associated with excessive muscle tension and relaxation. A simple set of verbal suggestions (e.g. 'Your left arm is becoming heavy and relaxed') made by the individual facilitating the relaxation can effectively reduce the level of muscle tension in the participant, with the same benefits, in the case of chronic pain, as outlined above.

Meditative techniques are also effective in reducing muscle tension, sympathetic activity and so on, incorporating breathing exercises and mental imagery. Saying a chosen word or phrase (not necessarily meaningful) with one's eyes closed, on exhalation, for example, can rapidly reduce the subjective tension felt by the patient. The simplest form this may take is simply saying the word 'one' repeatedly on exhalation while focusing attention on positive bodily sensations (warmth and so on). Some practice is required, since attention usually wanders in early sessions, and each session should last approximately half an hour. More active, positive mental imagery may also be incorporated in this kind of technique, whereby the patient imagines a personal, chosen image associated with positive, relaxing emotions (e.g. sitting by a stream). Those who advocate pure meditative techniques encourage the patient to focus entirely on the chosen repetitive phrase at the expense of all other thoughts, although this may not be attractive to some patients. In particular, maintaining this very narrow focus for long periods can result in unusual, and occasionally unpleasant, sensations of dissociation.

One final category of techniques provides the patient with physiological data regarding an index that is considered central to their subjective tension. Heart rate data, for example, can be amplified or presented visually so that the patient may use this 'biofeedback' to determine when the relaxation method being used is being successful. Other forms of biofeedback exist, including muscle tension data, measured by an electromyogram, and cortical arousal data, measured by an electroencephalogram. While biofeedback is effective, it requires expensive equipment that may appear rather impersonal and threatening to the patient. The feedback provided serves to reinforce the changes which result from whichever method of relaxation is adopted, but benefits are often no greater than those associated with simple, unreinforced relaxation methods. This may be because the parameters of interest (heart rate, for example) provide us with a degree of natural, internal biofeedback. The only area where there is evidence that biofeedback is more effective than simple relaxation is in the case of electromyogram feedback of muscle tension data in cases of localized muscle tension (e.g. tension headache).

Potential problems

Relaxation techniques have been shown to be particularly effective in cases of chronic headache and chronic low back pain. The different techniques all appear to be of equal effectiveness, and the choice should be driven by what the patient is most comfortable with. Expense considerations may also be important: Biofeedback is far more expensive than other forms of relaxation, but does not seem to provide much, if any, additional benefit except in a few specific cases. Moreover, because of the degree of intervention required by the individual facilitating biofeedback techniques there is a danger of excessive passivity on the part of the patient. One highly important feature of most relaxation techniques is that they encourage patients to take responsibility for their condition and its management.

Actual potential problems are few, although care should be taken after a relaxation session since one of the understandable consequences of such an intervention is a period of drowsiness or even sleep immediately after the session.

Hypnosis

The majority of adults, although by no means all, are hypnotizable, and the history of hypnosis is certainly a long one if, by hypnosis, one includes trance states, which are a common feature of most religions. It is only recently, however, that hypnosis has acquired a degree of medical respectability, with a variety of courses now available specifically for medical and health professionals.

The slow acceptance of hypnosis into mainstream medicine is to a large degree the result of a distorted popular image of hypnosis as a means of entertainment. Although around three-quarters of adults are hypnotizable, very few are suggestible to the degree that will result in them performing otherwise embarrassing acts in front of an audience. Moreover, a hypnotized individual is not at the mercy of the hypnotist but, rather, very relaxed and focusing exclusively on what the hypnotist is saying at the expense of other, extraneous stimuli. The individual is still conscious and able to exert his or her free will at any time if asked to do something they are unwilling to do. It is important to overcome these misconceptions before initiating a course of hypnosis in, for example, a chronic pain patient. It should be explained to the patient that the subjective unpleasantness of painful sensations is exacerbated by focusing on the pain.[2,3] Hypnotic suggestion may serve to distract the patient from the painful sensations, thereby improving subjective comfort.

Responsiveness

As stated above, roughly three-quarters of the adult population is hypnotizable, although it is impossible to predict in advance who will be. Stage hypnotists select those who are to appear on stage from a much larger, unseen group of volunteers, the majority of whom do not fit the hypnotist's criterion of extreme responsiveness to hypnotic suggestions. In hypnotherapy the most important considerations are the willingness of the patient to attempt hypnotic induction and the trust and confidence which the patient has in the individual who will be facilitating the hypnotic suggestion. The only personality trait which has been consistently found to be important is, unsurprisingly, the ability to maintain relatively high levels of concentration for a moderate length of time. Interestingly, hypnotic suggestion is often relatively easy in children because of children's ability to focus their concentration on single objects of interest for long periods.

Methods of induction

The induction of hypnosis is not complicated, although training on a course organized by a recognized body is, of course, important. The first step is to focus the attention of the patient (e.g. the swinging pocket watch of hypnotic folklore). A visual or auditory focus may be used, and this is followed by a period of relaxation and increasingly deep breathing. Mild suggestions may then be made to determine the extent to which the patient is hypnotizable (e.g. 'Your arm is getting lighter'). If the patient is sufficiently hypnotizable the course of sessions may be continued, using suggestions which encourage pain-incompatible imagery, until the patient is able to attain the same state themself by means of the same relaxation techniques.

Potential problems

Suggesting the use of hypnosis carries with it an implicit assumption, at least in the minds of some, that this means that the pain which it is used to manage is not 'real'. This misconception, and the allied one that such a technique must mean that the pain has no physical basis, is particularly damaging in the case of chronic pain, where patients may often be increasingly concerned that their problem is not taken sufficiently seriously.

A further potential problem is the passivity associated with hypnosis. For this reason it is important to maintain a degree of awareness in the patients regarding the procedures which are being followed, so that the patients may eventually be able to facilitate self-hypnosis themselves. To do this the patients must be aware of the stages in the hypnotic suggestion which are followed by the individual facilitating the trance state, so that these may be repeated later. Often tape recordings of hypnotic sessions are given to the patient to enable the patient to facilitate self-hypnosis elsewhere. These may be standardized recordings, or may be a recording of the actual sessions attended by the patient.

Conclusion

The advantages of hypnosis and relaxation techniques are their efficacy, at least in some patients, and the lack of side-effects. Moreover, if sufficient care is taken, these techniques may actually encourage the patient to take control of their condition and its management, with attendant improvements in psychosocial adjustment and well-being. The exact mechanisms which underlie the benefits of relaxation and hypnosis remain unclear, in particular in the case of hypnosis. Interestingly, the two appear to operate in quite different ways; that is, the effects of hypnotic suggestion on pain cannot be explained by the level of relaxation achieved by the hypnotized patient. Relaxation appears to reduce pain unpleasantness rather than pain intensity,[4] while hypnotic suggestion has the reverse effect, reducing levels of pain intensity rather than unpleasantness. More research is required to determine the mechanisms underlying the benefits of hypnotic analgesia if it is to become widely accepted. It is likely that hypnotic analgesia works in a variety of ways (e.g. by reducing the emotional component of pain, by reducing awareness of painful stimuli, by activating spinal anti-nociceptive mechanisms, and so on),[5] so that the nature of the hypnotic suggestion used may be tailored to the needs of the individual patient.

Summary
- Both relaxation and hypnotic suggestion represent simple methods of pain management, free from side-effects.
- These methods can readily be used in conjunction with other, more traditional, means of pain management.
- These methods can, in addition, be used to encourage self-reliance on the part of the patient, further improving rehabilitation.
- The benefits of these methods vary in a way which reflects the multi-dimensional nature of pain (e.g. emotional as well as sensory components).
- Evidence is emerging to suggest mechanisms which may underlie these techniques, which is valuable in encouraging their wider use.
- Misconceptions, in particular regarding the nature of hypnotic suggestion, must be dispelled to ensure the patient is happy to try these techniques.

References

1. Gatchel, R. J. and Turk, R. C. (eds) (1996) *Psychological Approaches to Pain Management: a Practitioner's Handbook.* New York: The Guilford Press.
2. Eccleston, C. Crombez, G., Aldrich, S. and Stannard, C. (1997) Attention and somatic awareness in chronic pain. *Pain*, 72, 209–15.

3. McCracken, L. M. (1997) 'Attention' to pain in persons with chronic pain: a behavioral approach. *Behavior Therapy*, 28, 271–84.
4. Dahlgren, L. A., Kurtz, R. M., Strube, M. J. and Malone, M. D. (1995) Differential effects of hypnotic suggestion on multiple dimensions of pain. *Journal of Pain and Symptom Management*, 10(6), 464–70.
5. Kiernan, B. D., Dane, J. R., Phillips, L. H. and Price, D. D. (1995) Hypnotic analgesia reduces R-III nociceptive reflex: further evidence concerning the multifactorial nature of hypnotic analgesia. *Pain*, 60, 39–47.

Index

Page numbers printed in **bold** type refer to figures; those in *italic* to tables